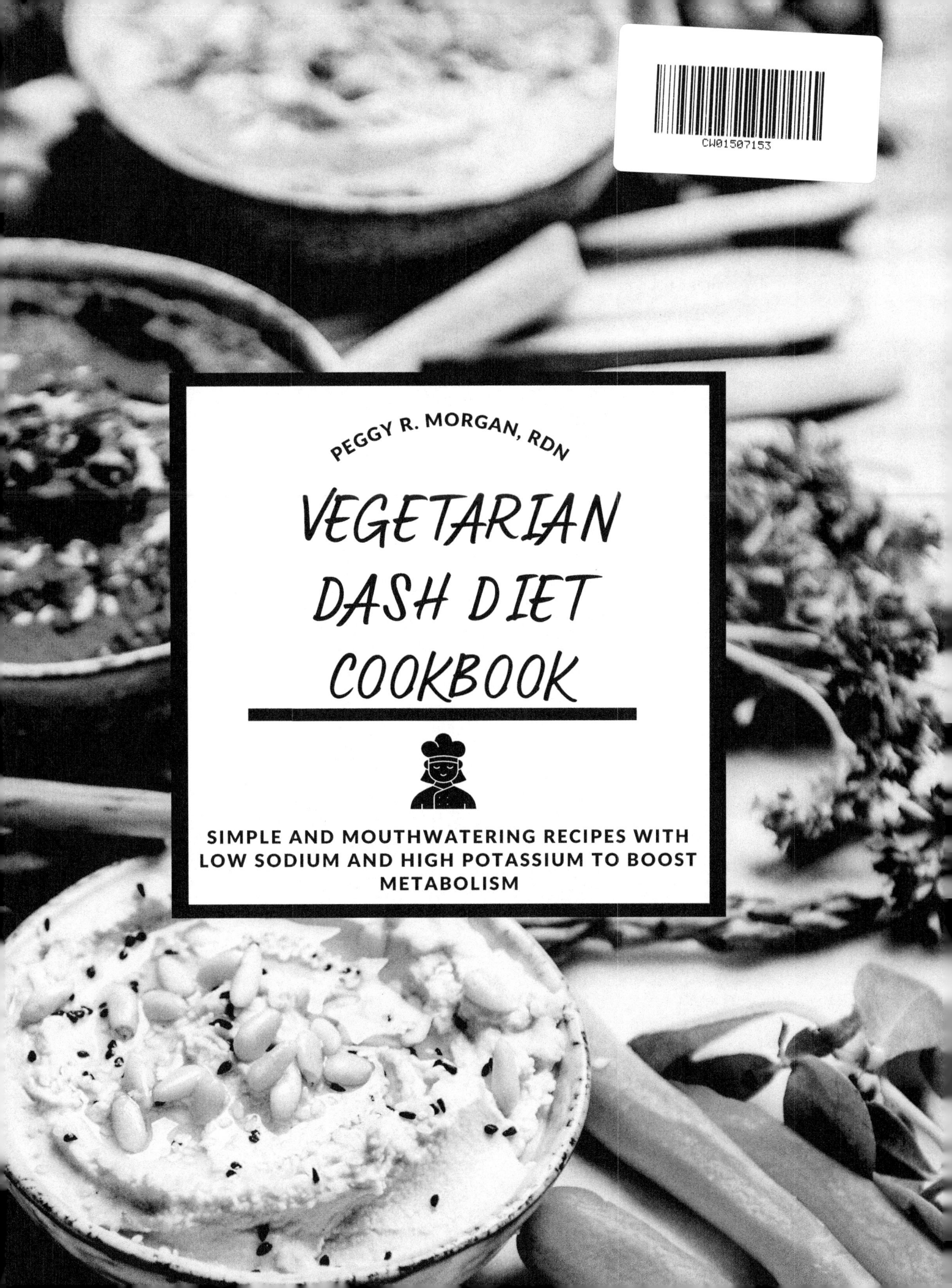

PEGGY R. MORGAN, RDN

VEGETARIAN DASH DIET COOKBOOK

SIMPLE AND MOUTHWATERING RECIPES WITH LOW SODIUM AND HIGH POTASSIUM TO BOOST METABOLISM

COPYRIGHT

DEDICATION

To all people who aspire for a healthy lifestyle via mindful eating, and to the power of plants in feeding both body and spirit. This book is dedicated to you, may it serve as a guiding light on your road to health and vitality.

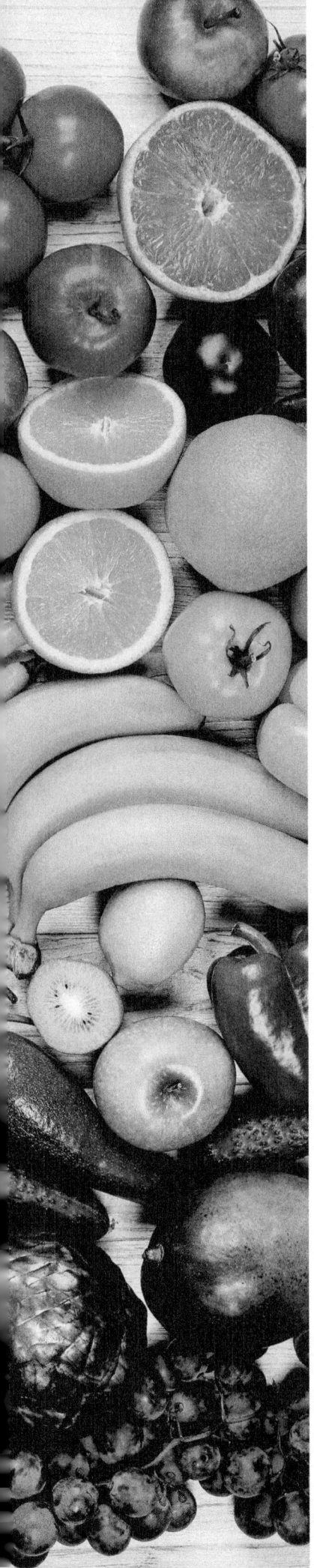

CONTENTS

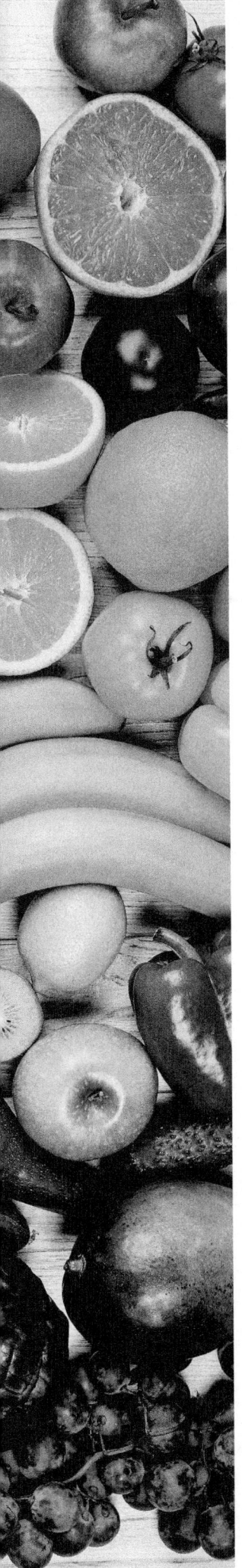

ACKNOWLEDGMENTS

I would like to show my deep thanks to everyone who helped with the making of this book. To my family and friends, thank you for your constant support and guidance throughout this journey. Your excitement for healthy eating has been truly amazing.

A special thank you to my loyal team, whose knowledge and advice helped bring this project to life. Your desire to support health through delicious, nutritious food has been priceless.

I am also deeply grateful to the people who have adopted the Vegetarian DASH Diet and are committed to bettering their health and well-being. Your excitement pushes me to continue sharing the joys of healthy cooking.

Last but not least, I convey my true thankfulness to the farmers, growers, and producers who develop the fresh, lively foods that make these recipes possible. Your hard work and commitment to sustainability improve our lives in countless ways.

Thank you, from the bottom of my heart, for being a part of this journey. May these meals bring you joy, health, and energy for years to come.

Peggy R. Morgan, RDN

INTRODUCTION TO VEGETARIAN DASH DIET

Say hello to the world of the Vegetarian DASH Diet—a mix of colorful plant-based food with the acclaimed Dietary Approaches to Stop Hypertension (DASH) diet! If you're here, you're likely interested in how to blend the concepts of the DASH Diet with a vegetarian lifestyle. But before we dig into the tasty dishes and practical ideas, let's start by explaining what it means to be a vegetarian.

Just imagine an era where vivid fruits, sharp veggies, sturdy grains, and nutritious legumes take pride of place on your plate. That's the core of vegetarianism. In its simplest form, a vegetarian is someone who abstains from ingesting meat, poultry, and fish. However, within the sphere of vegetarianism, there are many varieties.

One such variety is veganism, when people not only omit meat, poultry, and fish from their diet but also eschew all animal products, including dairy, eggs, and honey. On the other hand, a vegetarian diet generally includes dairy and eggs, making it more flexible for individuals who prefer to embrace plant-based eating while still enjoying certain animal-derived goods.

Now, consider the extensive array of tastes and sensations that may be weaved into a vegetarian perspective to the DASH diet. By combining the principles of DASH—known for its capacity to decrease blood pressure and promote heart health—with the wealth of plant-based goodness, we uncover a world of creative options that feed both body and spirit.

In this book, you'll uncover a treasure mine of 50 delectable and heart-healthy dishes painstakingly developed to comply with the Vegetarian DASH Diet. From invigorating breakfast bowls to delicious soups and salads, nutritious main meals to nourishing side dishes, and delectable snacks to decadent sweet treats, each recipe is meant to tickle your taste buds while supporting your health objectives.

But before we go into the cooking space, we're going to review the principles of the Vegetarian DASH Diet. We'll reveal the major concepts of the DASH diet, the advantages of adopting a vegetarian approach, and why maintaining a mix of low-sodium and high-potassium meals is vital for maximizing health. Plus, I'll give practical strategies for success and highlight key items and kitchen gear to keep on hand.

To make things even more easy, I've provided three weeks of modeling meal plans along with a matching grocery list for each week. Whether or not you're a seasoned vegetarian or beginning this lifestyle for the first time, these meal plans will serve as a guide to tasty, healthful eating.

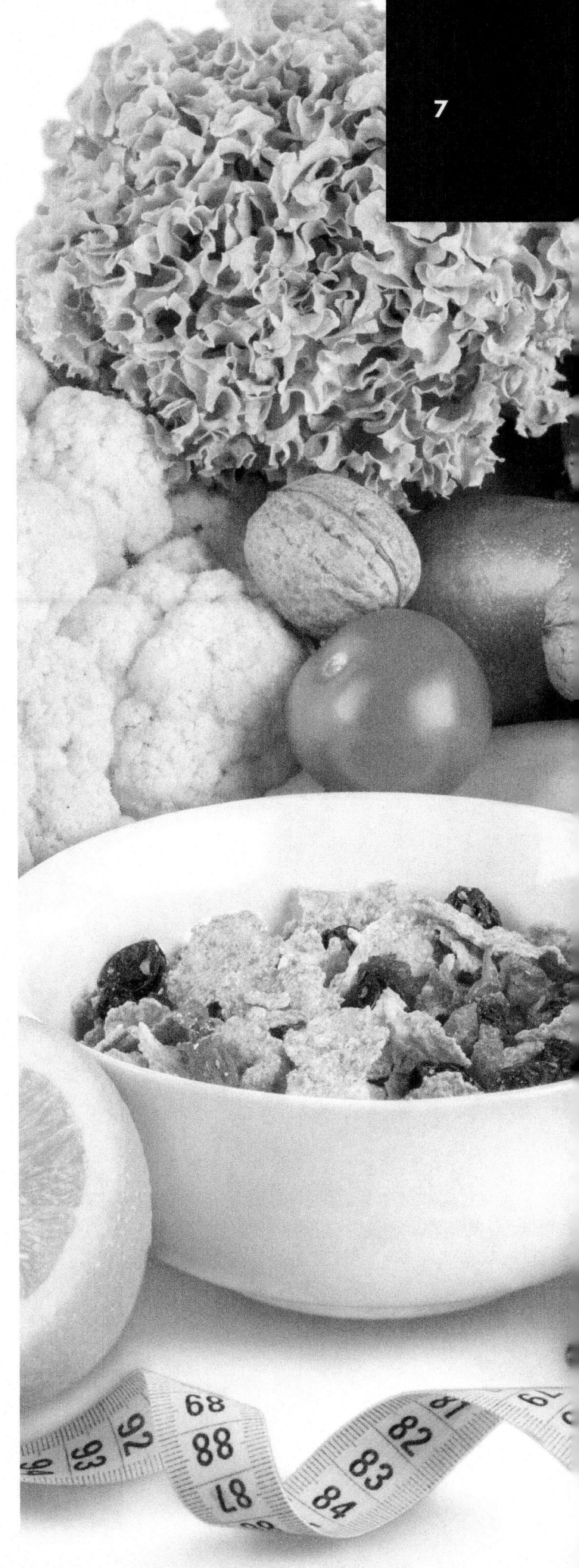

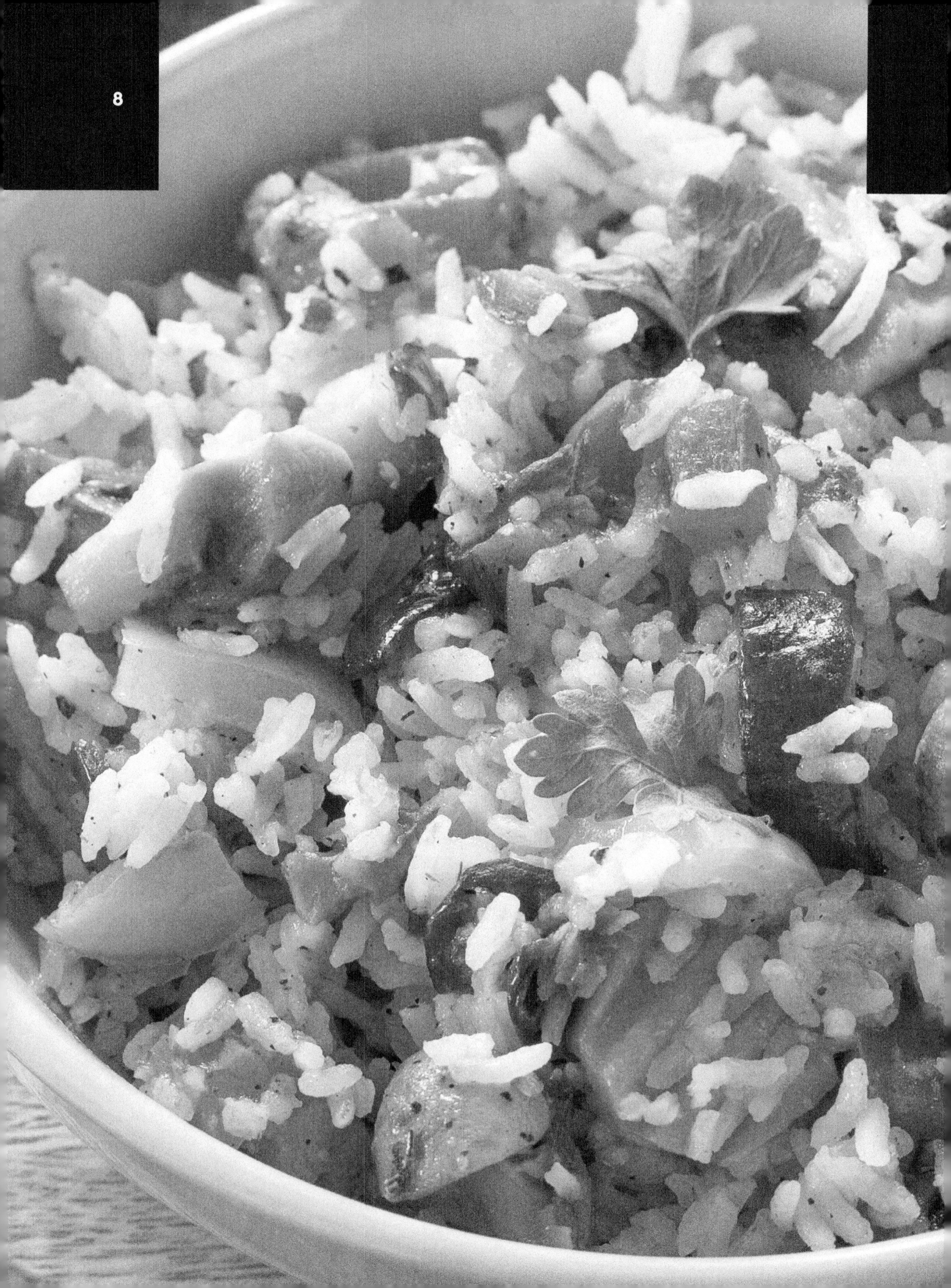

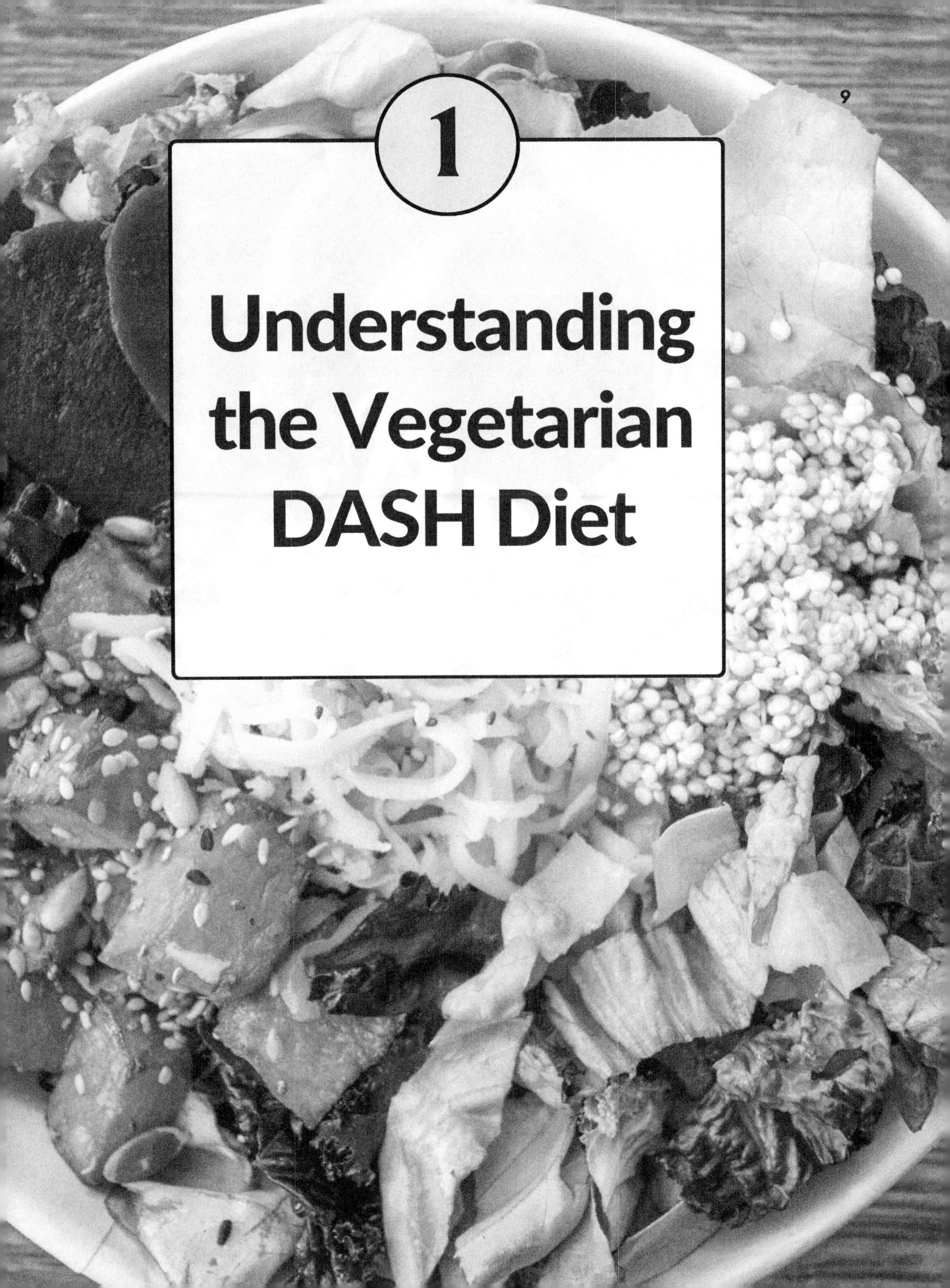

1

Understanding the Vegetarian DASH Diet

What is the DASH Diet?

DASH stands for **Dietary Approaches to Stop Hypertension**. But what does it truly mean? Well, it's a food plan particularly developed to help control and prevent high blood pressure, or hypertension. Developed by the National Institutes of Health (NIH), the DASH plan wasn't originally meant to be a weight-loss plan, but rather a means to address the rising worry of hypertension, a key risk factor for heart disease and stroke.

So, how does it work? The DASH Diet emphasizes eating enough of fruits, vegetables, whole grains, and lean meats while reducing meals rich in saturated fats, cholesterol, and salt. It's rich in minerals like potassium, magnesium, and fiber, which are proven to boost heart health and decrease blood pressure. By concentrating on these nutrient-dense foods and limiting salt consumption, the DASH Diet helps to support overall cardiovascular health.

The DASH Diet acquired popularity via numerous landmark studies, notably the DASH-Sodium research, which revealed the considerable blood pressure-lowering benefits of limiting salt consumption while following the DASH eating plan. Since then, other studies have further proven its usefulness in decreasing blood pressure and improving other aspects of cardiovascular health.

One of the amazing things about the DASH Diet is its versatility. It's not a one-size-fits-all method but rather a framework that can be modified to varied dietary tastes and lifestyles. Whether you're a meat-eater, vegetarian, or vegan, you can customize the DASH Diet to meet your requirements while still enjoying its health advantages.

In recent years, the DASH Diet has gained appeal beyond its initial emphasis on hypertension, with many individuals adopting it as a means to boost general health and well-being. Its focus on whole, nutrient-rich foods resonates with the principles of mindful eating and sustainable nutrition, making it a practical option for people aiming to feed their bodies and promote long-term health.

So, whether you want to control hypertension, enhance heart health, or just adopt a more wholesome attitude to eating, the DASH Diet provides a scientifically-backed route to greater health. It's not just a diet; it's a lifestyle that values tasty, healthy meals that feed your body and nurture the inner you.

Benefits of a Vegetarian Approach

"Why should I choose a Vegetarian approach to the DASH Diet?" Let's discover the myriad of perks waiting for you.

1. Heart Health: A Vegetarian DASH Diet offers a significant focus on entire plant foods such as fruits, vegetables, whole grains, legumes, nuts, and seeds. These foods are naturally low in saturated fat and cholesterol, which are recognized factors for heart disease. By adopting a vegetarian approach, you're preparing your food to promote cardiovascular health, minimizing your risk of heart disease and stroke.

2. Decrease Blood Pressure: The DASH Diet is recognized for its ability to decrease blood pressure, and a vegetarian twist further increases this benefit. Plant-based meals are rich in potassium, magnesium, and fiber, all of which play vital roles in managing blood pressure levels. By concentrating on plant foods, you're supplying your body with the nutrition it needs to maintain good blood pressure, without the extra salt frequently found in animal products.

3. Weight Management: Vegetarian diets tend to be lower in calories and richer in fiber compared to omnivore diets. This combination may improve weight control attempts by enhancing feelings of fullness and pleasure, lowering the probability of overeating. Additionally, plant-based meals are often less energy-dense than animal goods, meaning you may enjoy bigger servings with fewer calories, making weight maintenance or weight reduction more realistic.

4. Improved Digestive Health: Plant-based diets are naturally high in dietary fiber, which plays a critical role in digestive health. Fiber helps to produce regular bowel movements, avoid constipation, and maintain a healthy gut microbiota. By integrating a mix of fruits, vegetables, whole grains, legumes, nuts, and seeds into your diet, you're supplying your digestive system with the fiber it needs to flourish.

5. Reduced Risk of Chronic Illnesses: Research has repeatedly demonstrated that vegetarian diets are connected with a decreased risk of chronic illnesses such as type 2 diabetes, certain malignancies, and metabolic syndrome. By concentrating on whole plant meals, you're flooding your body with a plethora of vitamins, minerals, antioxidants, and phytonutrients that act synergistically to defend against illness and promote general health and longevity.

6. Environmental Sustainability: Choosing a vegetarian approach to the DASH Diet may also have good effects on the environment. Plant-based diets often have a reduced environmental impact compared to diets heavy in animal products. By limiting your intake of meat and dairy, you're helping to save water, decrease greenhouse gas emissions, and maintain natural ecosystems.

7. Longevity and Anti-Aging Advantages: Plant-based diets have been connected with longevity and anti-aging advantages owing to their nutrient-rich composition and protective effects against chronic illnesses. The amount of antioxidants present in fruits, vegetables, and other plant foods may assist in counteracting oxidative stress and inflammation, which are significant factors in aging and age-related disorders. By selecting plant-based meals, you're investing in your long-term health and well-being, increasing energy and resilience as you age.

8. Ethical Issues: For many people, choosing a Vegetarian DASH Diet extends beyond health and involves ethical issues connected to animal welfare. By opting to forego meat, poultry, and fish, you're aligning your dietary choices with ideals of compassion, generosity, and respect for all living creatures. This ethical component adds a deeper layer of significance to your dietary choices, building a feeling of connection with the environment around you and supporting a more sustainable and humane way of life.

By adopting plant-based foods and integrating them into the framework of the DASH Diet, you can feed your health, preserve the earth, and encourage a more compassionate way of eating and living.

Key Principles of the DASH Diet

The fundamental concepts of the DASH Diet are anchored in strong nutrition research and seek to increase heart health, decrease blood pressure, and improve general well-being. As we dig into these concepts, it's crucial to notice that they effortlessly fit with the beliefs and purposes of vegetarianism, making the Vegetarian DASH Diet a strong way to feed your body and safeguard your heart health.

1. Emphasize Fruits and Veggies: Aim to fill half of your plate with a variety of colorful fruits and veggies at each meal. These plant-based meals are rich in critical vitamins, minerals, antioxidants, and dietary fiber, which play a significant role in maintaining heart health, controlling blood pressure, and improving overall vitality.

2. Prioritize Whole Grains: Choose whole grains such as brown rice, quinoa, barley, oats, and whole wheat above refined grains like white rice and white bread. Whole grains are plentiful in fiber, which helps to decrease cholesterol levels, balance blood sugar, and maintain a healthy weight.

3. Include Lean Protein Sources: While standard DASH Diet guidelines include lean meats and poultry, vegetarians may acquire their protein from plant-based sources such as legumes (beans, lentils, chickpeas), tofu, tempeh, edamame, seitan, nuts, seeds, and dairy products (if lacto-vegetarian). These protein sources supply vital amino acids required for muscle upkeep, repair, and general health.

4. Limit Saturated Fat and Trans Fat: Opt for heart-healthy fats found in sources like avocados, almonds, seeds, olive oil, and fatty fish (for pescatarians) while reducing consumption of saturated and trans fats. Saturated fats, mostly found in animal products and processed diets, may boost LDL cholesterol levels and increase the risk of heart disease. Trans fats, frequently found in fried meals and baked products, have been related to inflammation and cardiovascular disorders.

5. Reduce Sodium Intake: Excessive sodium intake may boost blood pressure and increase the risk of heart disease. Aim to decrease sodium consumption by selecting fresh, whole foods over processed and packaged meals, which generally include high amounts of added salt. Flavor your foods using herbs, spices, citrus juices, and vinegar instead of depending on salt for flavor.

6. Moderate Alcohol Consumption: If you prefer to drink alcohol, do it in moderation. For most people, this implies up to one drink per day for women and up to two drinks per day for men. However, it's crucial to be cautious of portion sizes and to emphasize low-risk drinking practices to reduce any negative health impacts.

By accepting these fundamental concepts of the DASH Diet and adjusting them to a vegetarian lifestyle, you may build a satisfying and heart-healthy eating pattern that promotes longevity, vigor, and general well-being.

The Importance of Low Sodium and High Potassium

In the area of the DASH Diet, where we encourage the intake of nutrient-dense foods to enhance heart health and reduce blood pressure, the balance between sodium and potassium plays a vital role. Let's look into why these two minerals are of essential significance and how they affect our health within the framework of a vegetarian diet.

Sodium

Sodium is a mineral that's typically found in salt (sodium chloride). While our bodies need a certain amount of salt to operate effectively, excessive ingestion may lead to detrimental health consequences, notably on blood pressure. High salt consumption is commonly connected with hypertension, a significant risk factor for cardiovascular disease.

For vegetarians, it's crucial to be cautious of sodium levels, particularly because many processed vegetarian meals may include hidden sources of salt. By limiting salt consumption, we can assist manage blood pressure, enhance cardiovascular health, and minimize the risk of chronic illnesses.

Potassium

Potassium is another key element that plays a significant function in sustaining heart health. It helps counterbalance the effects of sodium by inducing vasodilation (the widening of blood vessels), which in turn helps reduce blood pressure. Potassium also maintains appropriate muscular function, neuronal transmission, and fluid equilibrium in the body.

Vegetarian diets may be naturally high in potassium since many plant-based foods are great providers of this mineral. Fruits like bananas, oranges, and avocados, as well as vegetables such as spinach, sweet potatoes, and tomatoes, are all high in potassium. By integrating these potassium-rich foods into our diet, we may help buffer the detrimental effects of salt and improve overall heart health.

Now, let's consider the practical ramifications of adding low-sodium and high-potassium meals into our vegetarian DASH Diet:

Reducing Sodium Intake: Opt for fresh, whole foods wherever feasible, since they tend to be lower in sodium compared to processed items. When cooking, flavor your dishes using herbs, spices, and citrus juices instead of depending excessively on salt. Read food labels carefully to uncover hidden sources of salt in packaged vegetarian items.

Increasing Potassium-Rich Foods: Make it a point to incorporate a range of potassium-rich foods in your vegetarian meals. Incorporate fruits, vegetables, legumes, nuts, and seeds into your regular diet to ensure you're fulfilling your potassium requirements. Experiment with various dishes and culinary approaches to make these nutrient-rich foods the star of your plate.

The daily recommendations for salt and potassium consumption might vary based on characteristics such as age, sex, and general health state. However, below are broad recommendations issued by health authorities:

1. Sodium: The American Heart Association (AHA) advises limiting salt consumption to no more than 2,300 milligrams (mg) per day for most persons. For patients with high blood pressure, cardiovascular disease, or certain other health concerns, the AHA advocates further decreasing salt consumption to 1,500 mg per day.

2. Potassium: The Dietary Guidelines for Americans suggest taking 4,700 mg of potassium per day for most individuals. However, it's vital to highlight that many individuals do not fulfill this guideline. Increasing potassium consumption via dietary sources, such as fruits, vegetables, legumes, nuts, and seeds, is suggested to improve general health and minimize the risk of hypertension and cardiovascular disease.

Establishing a balance between these two minerals is crucial to supporting heart health and decreasing blood pressure.

Tips for Success on the Vegetarian DASH Diet

1. Embrace Assortment: One of the keys to success on the Vegetarian DASH Diet is to embrace a broad range of plant-based meals. Aim to incorporate a rainbow of fruits and veggies in your meals to guarantee you're receiving a wide assortment of nutrients. Experiment with various grains, legumes, nuts, and seeds to make your meals new and enjoyable.

2. Focus on Whole Foods: When preparing your meals, consider entire, minimally processed foods. These include foods like fresh fruits and vegetables, whole grains, legumes, nuts, and seeds. Whole foods are rich in nutrients and fiber, which are crucial for maintaining general health and satiety.

3. Mind Your Portions: While plant-based meals are often fewer in calories compared to animal products, portion management is still vital for maintaining a healthy weight and attaining maximum health. Be aware of portion sizes, particularly when it comes to higher-calorie items like nuts, seeds, and avocados.

4. Balance Your Plate: Aim to prepare balanced meals that contain a mix of carbs, protein, and healthy fats. Fill half your plate with non-starchy veggies, a quarter with whole grains or starchy vegetables, and a quarter with protein-rich foods like beans, tofu, tempeh, or lentils. Add a source of healthy fat, such as avocado or olive oil, to finish out your meal.

5. Watch Your salt consumption: One of the fundamental components of the DASH Diet is lowering salt consumption to help control blood pressure. While many vegetarian meals are naturally low in sodium, it's still necessary to be cautious of added salt in packaged and processed foods, as well as in handmade recipes. Experiment with herbs, spices, citrus, and vinegar to add flavor to your dishes without depending on salt.

6. Target Potassium-Rich Foods: Potassium serves a critical function in controlling blood pressure and maintaining heart health. To enhance your potassium intake, add lots of potassium-rich foods to your diet, such as bananas, sweet potatoes, spinach, tomatoes, and beans. These items not only improve the taste and nutrients of your meals but also assist regulate salt levels in the body.

7. Stay Hydrated: Adequate hydration is crucial for general health and well-being. Make sure to drink lots of water throughout the day, particularly if you're eating a high-fiber diet. Herbal teas, flavored water, and coconut water are additional delightful choices to help you remain hydrated.

8. Plan and Prep Ahead: Set yourself up for success by planning and preparing your meals ahead of time. Spend some time each week preparing a meal plan, grocery shopping, and prepping items. Having nutritious meals and snacks readily accessible makes it simpler to keep to your nutritional objectives, especially on hectic days.

By adopting these guidelines into your lifestyle, you'll be well on your way to success on the Vegetarian DASH Diet. Remember, minor adjustments build up over time, so be patient with yourself and celebrate your success along the way.

Essential Ingredients and Kitchen Tools

Essential Ingredients

As you commence on your path with the Vegetarian DASH Diet, it's crucial to fill your pantry with healthful products that will form the basis of your meals. Here's a summary of some crucial items you'll want to have on hand:

Whole Grains: Quinoa, brown rice, oats, barley, millet, whole wheat pasta, and bulgur are good sources of fiber, which assists in digestion and helps manage blood sugar levels.

Legumes: Beans, lentils, chickpeas, and split peas are rich in protein, fiber, and vital minerals including iron and folate. They're flexible ingredients that may be used in soups, stews, salads, and even vegetarian burgers.

Fresh Produce: Load up on a variety of fruits and veggies, aiming for a colorful mix to ensure you're receiving a broad spectrum of vitamins, minerals, and antioxidants. Leafy greens like spinach, kale, and Swiss chard are especially rich in potassium, while berries and citrus fruits give a boost of vitamin C.

Nuts and Seeds: Incorporate heart-healthy fats and protein into your diet with nuts and seeds such as almonds, walnuts, chia seeds, flaxseeds, and hemp seeds. Sprinkle them over salads, yogurt, or cereal for additional crunch and nutrients.

Dairy and Plant-Based Alternatives: Opt for low-fat or non-fat dairy products like Greek yogurt, milk, and cheese. If you're following a vegan diet, pick fortified plant-based options such as almond milk, soy yogurt, and cashew cheese to guarantee you're fulfilling your calcium and vitamin D requirements.

Herbs and Spices: Enhance the taste of your foods without adding excessive salt by using a range of herbs and spices. Stock up on staples like garlic, onion, turmeric, cumin, paprika, basil, parsley, and cilantro to give depth and complexity to your recipes.

Kitchen Tools

In addition to filling your pantry with healthful products, having the correct kitchen utensils may make dinner preparation a breeze. Here are some crucial things to consider adding to your culinary arsenal:

High-Quality Chef's Knife: A sharp, multifunctional chef's knife is important for chopping, slicing, and dicing fruits, vegetables, and herbs with accuracy and simplicity.

Cutting Board: Invest in a robust cutting board made of wood or plastic to preserve your counters and offer a solid surface for food preparation.

Blender or Food Processor: Whether you're whipping up smoothies, pureeing soups, or preparing homemade sauces and dips, a blender or food processor may save you time and work in the kitchen.

Vegetable Spiralizer: Transform everyday veggies like zucchini, carrots, and sweet potatoes into noodles or ribbons for a fun and unique spin on typical pasta recipes.

Non-Stick Cookware: Invest in a set of high-quality non-stick pots and pans to avoid the need for extra oils and fats while cooking. Look for choices that are devoid of hazardous chemicals like PFOA and PFOS.

Steamer Basket: Steam your veggies to retain their nutrients and natural tastes while keeping their brilliant colors and crisp textures.

By filling your kitchen with these key goods and equipment, you'll be well-equipped to begin your Vegetarian DASH Diet journey with confidence and creativity.

Sample 3-Week Meal Plan

WEEK ONE

MONDAY

Breakfast: Peanut Butter Banana Overnight Oats
Mid-Morning: Greek Yogurt Parfait with Granola and Fresh Fruit
Lunch: Chickpea and Vegetable Stew
Snack: Mango Salsa with Baked Tortilla Chips
Dinner: Eggplant Parmesan with Whole Wheat Pasta
Dessert: Raspberry Almond Thumbprint Cookies
Beverage: Blueberry Lavender Lemonade

TUESDAY

Breakfast: Blueberry Almond Overnight Oats
Mid-Morning: Spinach and Artichoke Dip with Whole Wheat Pita Chips
Lunch: Black Bean and Sweet Potato Enchiladas
Snack: Mango Coconut Nice Cream
Dinner: Lentil and Vegetable Curry
Dessert: Pistachio and Cranberry Bark
Beverage: Cucumber Mint Cooler

WEDNESDAY

Breakfast: Whole Wheat Pancakes with Mixed Berries
Mid-Morning: Hummus with Crudites
Lunch: Quinoa and Vegetable Chowder
Snack: Carrot Cake Energy Bites
Dinner: Veggie Stir-Fry with Cashews
Dessert: Banana-Oat Cookies
Beverage: Kale Pineapple Smoothie

THURSDAY

Breakfast: Mushroom and Tomato Omelette
Mid-Morning: Baked Sweet Potato Fries with Chipotle Aioli
Lunch: Lentil Shepherd's Pie with Mashed Cauliflower Topping
Snack: Mixed Berry Crisp with Oat Topping
Dinner: Vegetable Paella with Saffron Rice
Dessert: Peanut Butter Banana Ice Cream
Beverage: Watermelon Basil Cooler

FRIDAY

Breakfast: Tofu Scramble Breakfast Burrito
Mid-Morning: Roasted Red Pepper and White Bean Dip with Whole Grain Pita Bread
Lunch: Sweet Potato and Kale Hash with Poached Eggs
Snack: Spicy Roasted Cauliflower Bites with Tahini Dipping Sauce
Dinner: Minestrone Soup with Whole Wheat Pasta
Dessert: Mango Coconut Nice Cream
Beverage: Cherry Almond Smoothie

SATURDAY

Breakfast: Veggie and Cheese Omelette
Mid-Morning: Cucumber Cups filled with Tzatziki and Diced Vegetables
Lunch: Spinach and Strawberry Salad with Balsamic Vinaigrette
Snack: Pistachio and Cranberry Bark
Dinner: Lentil and Vegetable Curry
Dessert: Carrot Cake Energy Bites
Beverage: Mango Lassi

SUNDAY

Breakfast: Tropical Paradise Smoothie Bowl
Mid-Morning: Caprese Salad with Fresh Basil
Lunch: Black Bean and Sweet Potato Soup
Snack: Roasted Red Pepper and White Bean Dip with Whole Grain Pita Bread
Dinner: Eggplant Parmesan with Whole Wheat Pasta
Dessert: Mixed Berry Crisp with Oat Topping
Beverage: Cranberry Ginger Sparkler

WEEK TWO

MONDAY

Breakfast: Peanut Butter Banana Overnight Oats
Mid-Morning: Greek Yogurt Parfait with Granola and Fresh Fruit
Lunch: Lentil and Vegetable Curry
Snack: Mango Salsa with Baked Tortilla Chips
Dinner: Veggie Stir-Fry with Cashews
Dessert: Raspberry Almond Thumbprint Cookies
Beverage: Blueberry Lavender Lemonade

TUESDAY

Breakfast: Tropical Paradise Smoothie Bowl
Mid-Morning: Hummus with Crudites
Lunch: Quinoa and Vegetable Chowder
Snack: Mango Salsa with Baked Tortilla Chips
Dinner: Lentil and Vegetable Curry
Dessert: Raspberry Almond Thumbprint Cookies
Beverage: Watermelon Basil Cooler

WEDNESDAY

Breakfast: Peanut Butter Banana Overnight Oats
Mid-Morning: Cucumber Cups filled with Tzatziki and Diced Vegetables
Lunch: Black Bean and Sweet Potato Enchiladas
Snack: Spinach and Artichoke Dip with Whole Wheat Pita Chips
Dinner: Eggplant Parmesan with Whole Wheat Pasta
Dessert: Mixed Berry Crisp with Oat Topping
Beverage: Blueberry Lavender Lemonade

THURSDAY

Breakfast: Veggie and Cheese Omelette
Mid-Morning: Mango Salsa with Baked Tortilla Chips
Lunch: Lentil Shepherd's Pie with Mashed Cauliflower Topping
Snack: Roasted Red Pepper and White Bean Dip with Whole Grain Pita Bread
Dinner: Sweet Potato and Kale Hash with Poached Eggs
Dessert: Banana-Oat Cookies
Beverage: Cranberry Ginger Sparkler

FRIDAY

Breakfast: Whole Wheat Pancakes with Mixed Berries
Mid-Morning: Greek Yogurt Parfait with Granola and Fresh Fruit
Lunch: Chickpea and Vegetable Stew
Snack: Carrot Cake Energy Bites
Dinner: Veggie Stir-Fry with Cashews
Dessert: Pistachio and Cranberry Bark
Beverage: Kale Pineapple Smoothie

SATURDAY

Breakfast: Blueberry Almond Overnight Oats
Mid-Morning: Mango Coconut Nice Cream
Lunch: Spinach and Strawberry Salad with Balsamic Vinaigrette
Snack: Baked Sweet Potato Fries with Chipotle Aioli
Dinner: Vegetable Paella with Saffron Rice
Dessert: Peanut Butter Banana Ice Cream
Beverage: Cucumber Mint Cooler

SUNDAY

Breakfast: Tofu Scramble Breakfast Burrito
Mid-Morning: Caprese Salad with Fresh Basil
Lunch: Minestrone Soup with Whole Wheat Pasta
Snack: Spicy Roasted Cauliflower Bites with Tahini Dipping Sauce
Dinner: Lentil and Vegetable Curry
Dessert: Carrot Cake Energy Bites
Beverage: Mango Lassi

WEEK THREE

MONDAY

Breakfast: Mushroom and Tomato Omelette
Mid-Morning: Pistachio and Cranberry Bark
Lunch: Black Bean and Sweet Potato Soup
Snack: Hummus with Crudites
Dinner: Eggplant Parmesan with Whole Wheat Pasta
Dessert: Mixed Berry Crisp with Oat Topping
Beverage: Cherry Almond Smoothie

TUESDAY

Breakfast: Veggie Stir-Fry with Cashews
Mid-Morning: Hummus with Crudites
Lunch: Chickpea and Vegetable Stew
Snack: Mango Coconut Nice Cream
Dinner: Black Bean and Sweet Potato Enchiladas
Dessert: Mixed Berry Crisp with Oat Topping
Beverage: Cherry Almond Smoothie

WEDNESDAY

Breakfast: Tofu Scramble Breakfast Burrito
Mid-Morning: Caprese Salad with Fresh Basil
Lunch: Lentil and Vegetable Curry
Snack: Spicy Roasted Cauliflower Bites with Tahini Dipping Sauce
Dinner: Eggplant Parmesan with Whole Wheat Pasta
Dessert: Mango Coconut Nice Cream
Beverage: Cucumber Mint Cooler

THURSDAY

Breakfast: Blueberry Almond Overnight Oats
Mid-Morning: Mango Lassi
Lunch: Black Bean and Sweet Potato Soup
Snack: Hummus with Crudites
Dinner: Veggie and Cheese Omelette
Dessert: Pistachio and Cranberry Bark
Beverage: Cherry Almond Smoothie

SATURDAY

Breakfast: Veggie and Cheese Omelette
Mid-Morning: Caprese Salad with Fresh Basil
Lunch: Chickpea and Vegetable Stew
Snack: Pistachio and Cranberry Bark
Dinner: Eggplant Parmesan with Whole Wheat Pasta
Dessert: Mixed Berry Crisp with Oat Topping
Beverage: Cranberry Ginger Sparkler

FRIDAY

Breakfast: Mushroom and Tomato Omelette
Mid-Morning: Baked Sweet Potato Fries with Chipotle Aioli
Lunch: Minestrone Soup with Whole Wheat Pasta
Snack: Mango Salsa with Baked Tortilla Chips
Dinner: Vegetable Paella with Saffron Rice
Dessert: Carrot Cake Energy Bites
Beverage: Cranberry Ginger Sparkler

SUNDAY

Breakfast: Tropical Paradise Smoothie Bowl
Mid-Morning: Hummus with Crudites
Lunch: Lentil and Vegetable Curry
Snack: Mango Salsa with Baked Tortilla Chips
Dinner: Sweet Potato and Kale Hash with Poached Eggs
Dessert: Banana-Oat Cookies
Beverage: Watermelon Basil Cooler

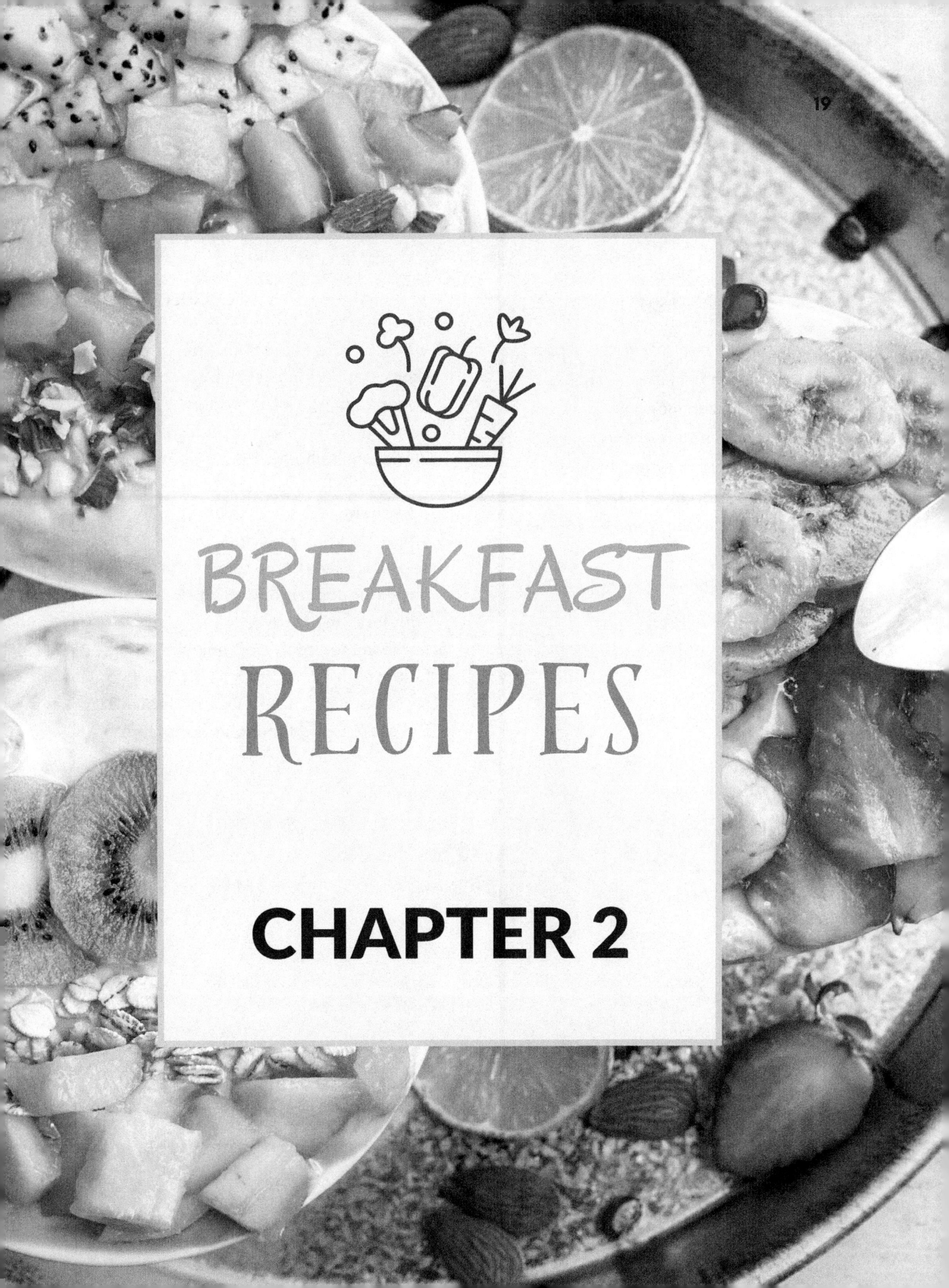

BREAKFAST RECIPES

CHAPTER 2

Tropical Paradise Smoothie Bowl

Servings: 2 Prep Time: 10 mins Cook Time: 0 min Total Time: 10 mins

Ingredients

2 ripe bananas, frozen and sliced

1 cup frozen pineapple chunks

1 cup frozen mango chunks

1/2 cup unsweetened coconut milk

1/4 cup plain Greek yogurt

1 tablespoon chia seeds

1 tablespoon unsweetened shredded coconut

1 tablespoon honey or maple syrup (optional, adjust to taste)

Fresh mint leaves for garnish

Procedures

1. In a blender, combine the frozen banana slices, pineapple chunks, mango chunks, coconut milk, Greek yogurt, chia seeds, and honey or maple syrup (if using).
2. Blend until smooth and creamy, adding more coconut milk if needed to reach your desired consistency.
3. Once blended, pour the smoothie into bowls.
4. Top each smoothie bowl with a sprinkle of unsweetened shredded coconut and garnish with fresh mint leaves.
5. Serve immediately and enjoy!
6. Serve with Fresh fruit slices (such as kiwi or strawberries), or granola or toasted coconut flakes for added crunch and texture

Nutritional Value (per serving): Calories: 250 Kcal, Carbohydrates: 48 g, Proteins: 5 g, Fats: 7 g, Sodium: 30 mg, Potassium: 550 mg, Fiber: 8 g, Sugar: 30 g

Veggie and Cheese Omelette

Servings: 2   Prep Time: 10 mins   Cook Time: 10 mins Total Time: 20 mins

Ingredients

4 large eggs
1/4 cup diced bell peppers (any color)
1/4 cup diced tomatoes
1/4 cup diced onions
1/4 cup chopped spinach
1/4 cup shredded low-fat cheese
1 tablespoon olive oil
1/2 teaspoon dried oregano
1/2 teaspoon dried basil
1/4 teaspoon black pepper

Procedures

1. In a bowl, beat the eggs until well combined.
2. Heat the olive oil in a non-stick skillet over medium heat.
3. Add the diced bell peppers, tomatoes, onions, and chopped spinach to the skillet. Sauté for 3-4 minutes until vegetables are tender.
4. Pour the beaten eggs over the sautéed vegetables in the skillet.
5. Sprinkle the shredded low-fat cheese evenly over the eggs.
6. Sprinkle the dried oregano, dried basil, and black pepper over the cheese.
7. Cook the omelette for 3-4 minutes or until the edges start to set.
8. Carefully flip the omelette using a spatula and cook for an additional 2-3 minutes until cooked through.
9. Once cooked, slide the omelette onto a plate and fold it in half.
10. Serve hot with whole grain toast or a side of fresh fruit.

Nutritional Value (per serving): Calories: 180 Kcal, Carbohydrates: 5 g, Proteins: 14 g, Fats: 11 g, Sodium: 250 mg, Potassium: 320 mg, Fiber: 2 g, Sugar: 2 g

Peanut Butter Banana Overnight Oats

Servings: 2   Prep Time: 5 mins   Total Time: 8 hours (plus chilling time)

Ingredients

1 cup rolled oats

1 cup unsweetened almond milk

2 tablespoons natural peanut butter

1 ripe banana, mashed

1 tablespoon chia seeds

1 tablespoon maple syrup or honey
(optional, adjust to taste)

1 teaspoon ground cinnamon

1/2 teaspoon vanilla extract

Pinch of nutmeg

Fresh berries or sliced banana, for
topping (optional)

Procedures

1. In a mixing bowl, combine rolled oats, almond milk, peanut butter, mashed banana, chia seeds, maple syrup (if using), cinnamon, vanilla extract, and nutmeg. Stir until well combined.
2. Divide the mixture evenly between two serving jars or containers with lids.
3. Cover the jars or containers and refrigerate overnight, or for at least 6-8 hours, to allow the oats to soften and flavors to meld.
4. Before serving, give the oats a good stir. If the mixture is too thick, you can add a splash of almond milk to reach your desired consistency.
5. Serve topped with fresh berries or sliced banana, if desired.

Nutritional Value (per serving): Calories: 320 Kcal, Carbohydrates: 42 g, Proteins: 9 g, Fats: 14 g, Sodium:

Blueberry Almond Overnight Oats

Servings: 2   Prep Time: 5 mins   Total Time: Overnight + 5 minutes

Ingredients

1 cup rolled oats

1 cup unsweetened almond milk

1/2 cup fresh blueberries

2 tablespoons almond butter

1 tablespoon maple syrup or honey
(optional, for sweetness)

1/2 teaspoon cinnamon

1/4 teaspoon nutmeg

1/4 teaspoon vanilla extract

Chopped almonds, for garnish

Fresh mint leaves, for garnish

Procedures

1. In a mixing bowl, combine the rolled oats, almond milk, almond butter, maple syrup (if using), cinnamon, nutmeg, and vanilla extract. Stir well to combine all ingredients evenly.
2. Gently fold in the fresh blueberries, ensuring they are evenly distributed throughout the mixture.
3. Divide the mixture evenly between two small jars or containers with lids.
4. Cover the jars or containers with lids and refrigerate overnight, or for at least 4 hours, to allow the oats to soften and absorb the flavors.
5. When ready to serve, remove the jars or containers from the refrigerator and give the oats a stir.
6. Garnish with chopped almonds and fresh mint leaves, if desired, before serving.

Nutritional Value (per serving): Calories: 280 Kcal, Carbohydrates: 37 g, Proteins: 8 g, Fats: 11 g, Sodium: 80 mg, Potassium: 280 mg, Fiber: 7 g, Sugar: 7 g

Mushroom and Tomato Omelette

Servings: 2   Prep Time: 10 mins   Cook Time: 10 mins Total Time: 20 mins

Ingredients

4 large eggs
1 cup sliced mushrooms
1 medium tomato, diced
1/4 cup chopped onion
1/4 teaspoon black pepper
1/4 teaspoon paprika
1/4 teaspoon dried thyme
1 tablespoon olive oil

Procedures

1. In a mixing bowl, beat the eggs until well blended. Stir in the black pepper, paprika, and dried thyme. Set aside.
2. Heat the olive oil in a non-stick skillet over medium heat.
3. Add the chopped onion to the skillet and sauté for 2-3 minutes until softened.
4. Add the sliced mushrooms to the skillet and cook for another 3-4 minutes until they begin to release their juices.
5. Stir in the diced tomatoes and continue to cook for 1-2 minutes until they are heated through.
6. Pour the beaten egg mixture over the vegetables in the skillet. Allow the eggs to cook undisturbed for a minute or two until the edges start to set.
7. Using a spatula, gently lift the edges of the omelette and tilt the skillet to let the uncooked egg flow underneath.
8. Continue cooking until the omelette is set but still slightly moist on top.
9. Carefully fold the omelette in half and cook for another 1-2 minutes until the eggs are fully cooked.
10. Slide the omelette onto a plate and serve hot.

Nutritional Value (per serving): Calories: 178 Kcal, Carbohydrates: 5.8 g, Proteins: 12.6 g, Fats: 11.8 g,

Tofu Scramble Breakfast Burrito

Servings: 2   Prep Time: 10 mins   Cook Time: 10 mins Total Time: 20 mins

Ingredients

1 block (14 oz) firm tofu, drained and crumbled

1 tablespoon olive oil

1/2 teaspoon turmeric powder

1/2 teaspoon paprika

1/2 teaspoon garlic powder

1/2 teaspoon onion powder

1/4 teaspoon ground black pepper

1/2 cup diced bell peppers (any color)

1/2 cup diced onions

1/2 cup diced tomatoes

2 large whole grain tortillas

1/2 avocado, sliced

Fresh cilantro, for garnish

Procedures

1. Heat olive oil in a skillet over medium heat. Add diced onions and bell peppers. Cook until softened, about 3-4 minutes.
2. Add crumbled tofu to the skillet. Sprinkle turmeric powder, paprika, garlic powder, onion powder, and black pepper over the tofu. Stir well to combine and cook for another 5-6 minutes until tofu is heated through and slightly golden.
3. Add diced tomatoes to the skillet and cook for an additional 1-2 minutes until heated through.
4. Warm the tortillas in a separate skillet or microwave for a few seconds until pliable.
5. Divide the tofu scramble mixture evenly between the tortillas. Top each with sliced avocado and fresh cilantro.
6. Roll up the tortillas into burritos, folding in the sides as you go.
7. Serve immediately and enjoy.

Nutritional Value (per serving): Calories: 320 Kcal, Carbohydrates: 25 g, Proteins: 15 g, Fats: 20 g, Sodium: 120 mg, Potassium: 580 mg, Fiber: 8 g, Sugar: 4 g

Whole Wheat Pancakes with Mixed Berries

Servings: 2   Prep Time: 10 mins   Cook Time: 10 mins   Total Time: 20 mins

Ingredients

1 cup whole wheat flour

1 tablespoon baking powder

1 tablespoon ground flaxseed (optional)

1 tablespoon maple syrup or agave nectar

1 cup almond milk or any non-dairy milk

1 tablespoon coconut oil, melted

1 teaspoon vanilla extract

1 cup mixed berries (such as strawberries, blueberries, raspberries)

Procedures

1. In a large mixing bowl, combine the whole wheat flour, baking powder, and ground flaxseed (if using). Mix well.
2. Add the maple syrup, almond milk, melted coconut oil, and vanilla extract to the dry ingredients. Stir until just combined. Be careful not to overmix; a few lumps are okay.
3. Heat a non-stick skillet or griddle over medium heat. Lightly grease with coconut oil or cooking spray.
4. Pour about 1/4 cup of batter onto the skillet for each pancake. Cook until bubbles form on the surface and the edges start to look set, about 2-3 minutes.
5. Flip the pancakes and cook for another 1-2 minutes, until golden brown and cooked through.
6. Serve the pancakes warm, topped with mixed berries.

Servings: 2 Prep Time: 10 mins Cook Time: 0 min   Total Time: 10 mins

Ingredients

1 cup Greek yogurt (unsweetened)

1/2 cup granola (unsweetened)

1/2 cup mixed fresh fruits (such as berries, sliced bananas, or chopped mangoes)

1 tablespoon honey or maple syrup (optional, for sweetness)

1/2 teaspoon ground cinnamon

Fresh mint leaves for garnish

Procedures

1. In a bowl or glass, layer half of the Greek yogurt at the bottom.
2. Sprinkle half of the granola on top of the yogurt layer.
3. Add half of the mixed fresh fruits on top of the granola.
4. Drizzle with honey or maple syrup if desired, for a touch of sweetness.
5. Repeat the layering process with the remaining yogurt, granola, and fresh fruits.
6. Sprinkle ground cinnamon over the top layer.
7. Garnish with fresh mint leaves for an extra burst of flavor.
8. Serve immediately and enjoy!

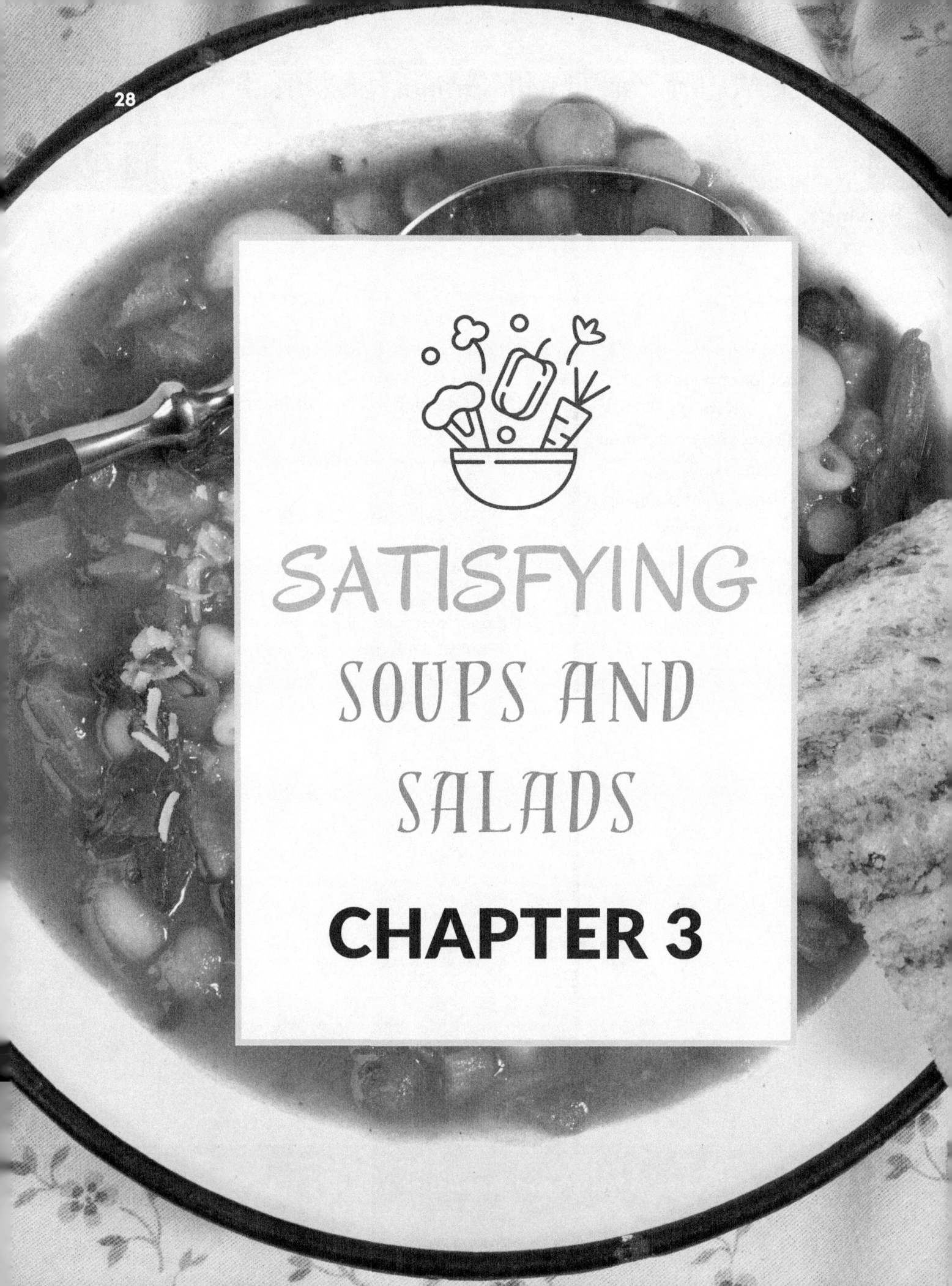

SATISFYING

SOUPS AND

SALADS

CHAPTER 3

Minestrone Soup with Whole Wheat Pasta

Servings: 2 Prep Time: 10 mins Cook Time: 20 mins Total Time: 30 mins

Ingredients

1 tablespoon olive oil

1 small onion, diced

2 cloves garlic, minced

1 carrot, diced

1 celery stalk, diced

1 small zucchini, diced

1 cup canned diced tomatoes (low-sodium)

4 cups vegetable broth (low-sodium)

1/2 cup whole wheat pasta shells

1 teaspoon dried basil

1/2 teaspoon dried oregano

1/2 teaspoon dried thyme

1 bay leaf

Freshly ground black pepper, to taste

1 cup chopped spinach or kale

1/4 cup chopped fresh parsley

Lemon wedges, for serving

Procedures

1. Heat olive oil in a large pot over medium heat. Add diced onion and garlic, and sauté until softened, about 3-4 minutes.
2. Add diced carrot, celery, and zucchini to the pot. Cook for another 5 minutes, stirring occasionally.
3. Pour in the canned diced tomatoes and vegetable broth. Bring to a boil.
4. Once boiling, add whole wheat pasta shells, dried basil, dried oregano, dried thyme, bay leaf, and freshly ground black pepper. Reduce heat to a simmer and cook for about 10-12 minutes, or until pasta is tender.
5. Stir in chopped spinach or kale and cook for an additional 2-3 minutes until wilted.
6. Remove the bay leaf from the soup. Taste and adjust seasoning if necessary.
7. Serve hot, garnished with chopped fresh parsley and lemon wedges on the side for squeezing over the soup.

Nutritional Value (per serving): Calories: 230 Kcal, Carbohydrates: 35 g, Proteins: 7 g, Fats: 8 g, Sodium: 290 mg, Potassium: 680 mg, Fiber: 8 g, Sugar: 6 g

Chickpea and Vegetable Stew

Servings: 2   Prep Time: 10 mins   Cook Time: 25 mins   Total Time: 35 mins

Ingredients

1 tablespoon olive oil

1 onion, diced

2 cloves garlic, minced

1 carrot, diced

1 celery stalk, diced

1 bell pepper, diced

1 can (15 ounces) chickpeas, drained and rinsed

1 can (14.5 ounces) diced tomatoes, undrained

2 cups vegetable broth

1 teaspoon paprika

1/2 teaspoon cumin

1/2 teaspoon dried thyme

1/2 teaspoon dried rosemary

1/4 teaspoon black pepper

2 cups spinach leaves, chopped

Fresh parsley, for garnish (optional)

Procedures

1. Heat the olive oil in a large pot over medium heat. Add the diced onion and cook until translucent, about 3-4 minutes.
2. Add the minced garlic, diced carrot, diced celery, and diced bell pepper to the pot. Cook, stirring occasionally, until the vegetables are slightly softened, about 5 minutes.
3. Stir in the drained and rinsed chickpeas, diced tomatoes (with their juices), vegetable broth, paprika, cumin, dried thyme, dried rosemary, and black pepper. Bring the mixture to a simmer.
4. Reduce the heat to low, cover the pot, and let the stew simmer for about 15 minutes to allow the flavors to meld together and the vegetables to become tender.
5. Stir in the chopped spinach leaves and cook for an additional 2-3 minutes until the spinach is wilted.
6. Taste and adjust seasoning if needed. Serve hot, garnished with fresh parsley if desired.

Nutritional Value (per serving): Calories: 240 Kcal, Carbohydrates: 35 g, Proteins: 10 g, Fats: 8 g, Sodium: 460 mg, Potassium: 820 mg, Fiber: 10 g, Sugar: 9 g

Quinoa and Vegetable Chowder

Servings: 2   Prep Time: 10 mins   Cook Time: 25 mins   Total Time: 35 mins

Ingredients

1/2 cup quinoa, rinsed

1 tablespoon olive oil

1/2 onion, diced

2 cloves garlic, minced

1 carrot, diced

1 celery stalk, diced

1/2 red bell pepper, diced

1/2 teaspoon paprika

1/2 teaspoon dried thyme

1/2 teaspoon dried rosemary

1/4 teaspoon black pepper

2 cups vegetable broth

1 cup water

1 cup spinach leaves, chopped

1/4 cup non-fat Greek yogurt
(optional, for garnish)

Fresh parsley, chopped (for garnish)

Procedures

1. In a medium-sized pot, heat the olive oil over medium heat. Add the diced onion, minced garlic, carrot, celery, and red bell pepper. Sauté for 5-7 minutes until the vegetables are softened.
2. Add the rinsed quinoa to the pot along with the paprika, dried thyme, dried rosemary, and black pepper. Stir to combine.
3. Pour in the vegetable broth and water, and bring the mixture to a boil. Once boiling, reduce the heat to low, cover, and simmer for 15-20 minutes, or until the quinoa is cooked through.
4. Once the quinoa is cooked, stir in the chopped spinach leaves and let them wilt for 2-3 minutes.
5. Remove the pot from the heat and ladle the chowder into bowls. If desired, top each serving with a dollop of non-fat Greek yogurt and a sprinkle of fresh parsley.
6. Serve hot and enjoy!

Nutritional Value (per serving): Calories: 270 Kcal, Carbohydrates: 41 g, Proteins: 10 g, Fats: 7 g, Sodium: 315 mg, Potassium: 635 mg, Fiber: 7 g, Sugar: 4 g

Black Bean and Sweet Potato Soup

Servings: 2   Prep Time: 10 mins   Cook Time: 25 mins Total Time: 35 mins

Ingredients

1 tablespoon olive oil

1 small onion, diced

2 cloves garlic, minced

1 teaspoon ground cumin

1/2 teaspoon chili powder

1/4 teaspoon smoked paprika

1 medium sweet potato, peeled and diced

1 (15 oz) can black beans, drained and rinsed

2 cups vegetable broth

1 cup water

1 tablespoon lime juice

Freshly ground black pepper, to taste

Chopped fresh cilantro, for garnish

Sliced avocado, for garnish

Procedures

1. In a large pot, heat the olive oil over medium heat. Add the diced onion and cook until softened, about 5 minutes.
2. Add the minced garlic, ground cumin, chili powder, and smoked paprika to the pot. Stir and cook for another 1-2 minutes until fragrant.
3. Add the diced sweet potato, black beans, vegetable broth, and water to the pot. Bring to a simmer and cook for 15-20 minutes, or until the sweet potatoes are tender.
4. Once the sweet potatoes are tender, use an immersion blender to blend the soup until smooth and creamy. Alternatively, transfer half of the soup to a blender and blend until smooth, then return it to the pot.
5. Stir in the lime juice and season with freshly ground black pepper, to taste.
6. Ladle the soup into bowls and garnish with chopped fresh cilantro and sliced avocado.

Nutritional Value (per serving): Calories: 260 Kcal, Carbohydrates: 42 g, Proteins: 10 g, Fats: 7 g, Sodium: 480 mg, Potassium: 820 mg, Fiber: 11 g, Sugar: 6 g

Spinach and Strawberry Salad with Balsamic Vinaigrette

Servings: 2   Prep Time: 10 mins   Cook Time: 0 min   Total Time: 10 mins

Ingredients

4 cups fresh spinach leaves, washed and dried

1 cup fresh strawberries, sliced

1/4 cup chopped walnuts

2 tablespoons balsamic vinegar

1 tablespoon extra virgin olive oil

1 teaspoon Dijon mustard

1/2 teaspoon dried oregano

1/2 teaspoon dried basil

Freshly ground black pepper, to taste

Procedures

1. In a large mixing bowl, combine the fresh spinach leaves and sliced strawberries.
2. In a small bowl, whisk together the balsamic vinegar, olive oil, Dijon mustard, dried oregano, and dried basil until well combined.
3. Drizzle the balsamic vinaigrette over the spinach and strawberry mixture and toss gently to coat.
4. Sprinkle the chopped walnuts over the salad.
5. Season with freshly ground black pepper to taste.
6. Serve immediately and enjoy!

Nutritional Value (per serving): Calories: 150 Kcal, Carbohydrates: 10 g, Proteins: 3 g, Fats: 11 g, Sodium: 5

Caprese Salad with Fresh Basil

Servings: 2   Prep Time: 10 mins   Cook Time: 0 min   Total Time: 10 mins

Ingredients

2 ripe tomatoes, sliced

4 oz fresh mozzarella cheese, sliced

1/4 cup fresh basil leaves

1 tablespoon extra virgin olive oil

1 tablespoon balsamic vinegar

1/2 teaspoon dried oregano

1/4 teaspoon black pepper

Procedures

1. Arrange the tomato and mozzarella slices alternately on a serving plate.
2. Tuck fresh basil leaves between the tomato and cheese slices.
3. In a small bowl, whisk together the extra virgin olive oil, balsamic vinegar, dried oregano, and black pepper.
4. Drizzle the dressing over the salad.
5. Serve immediately and enjoy!

Nutritional Value (per serving): Calories: 180 Kcal, Carbohydrates: 7 g, Proteins: 9 g, Fats: 13 g, Sodium: 60 mg, Potassium: 260 mg, Fiber: 2 g, Sugar: 5 g

Servings: 2   Prep Time: 10 mins   Cook Time: 0 min   Total Time: 10 mins

Ingredients

4 cups arugula, washed and dried

1 ripe pear, thinly sliced

1/4 cup walnuts, chopped

2 tablespoons olive oil

1 tablespoon Dijon mustard

1 tablespoon apple cider vinegar

1 teaspoon honey (optional, for sweetness)

1/4 teaspoon black pepper

1/4 teaspoon dried thyme

1/4 teaspoon dried oregano

Procedures

1. In a large salad bowl, combine the arugula, sliced pear, and chopped walnuts.
2. In a small mixing bowl, whisk together the olive oil, Dijon mustard, apple cider vinegar, honey (if using), black pepper, dried thyme, and dried oregano until well combined.
3. Drizzle the Dijon vinaigrette over the salad ingredients in the bowl.
4. Toss the salad gently to coat everything evenly with the dressing.
5. Divide the salad into two serving plates or bowls.
6. Serve immediately and enjoy the refreshing flavors of this arugula and pear salad.

Nutritional Value (per serving): Calories: 180 Kcal, Carbohydrates: 14 g, Proteins: 2 g, Fats: 14 g, Sodium: 45 mg, Potassium: 210 mg, Fiber: 4 g, Sugar: 7 g

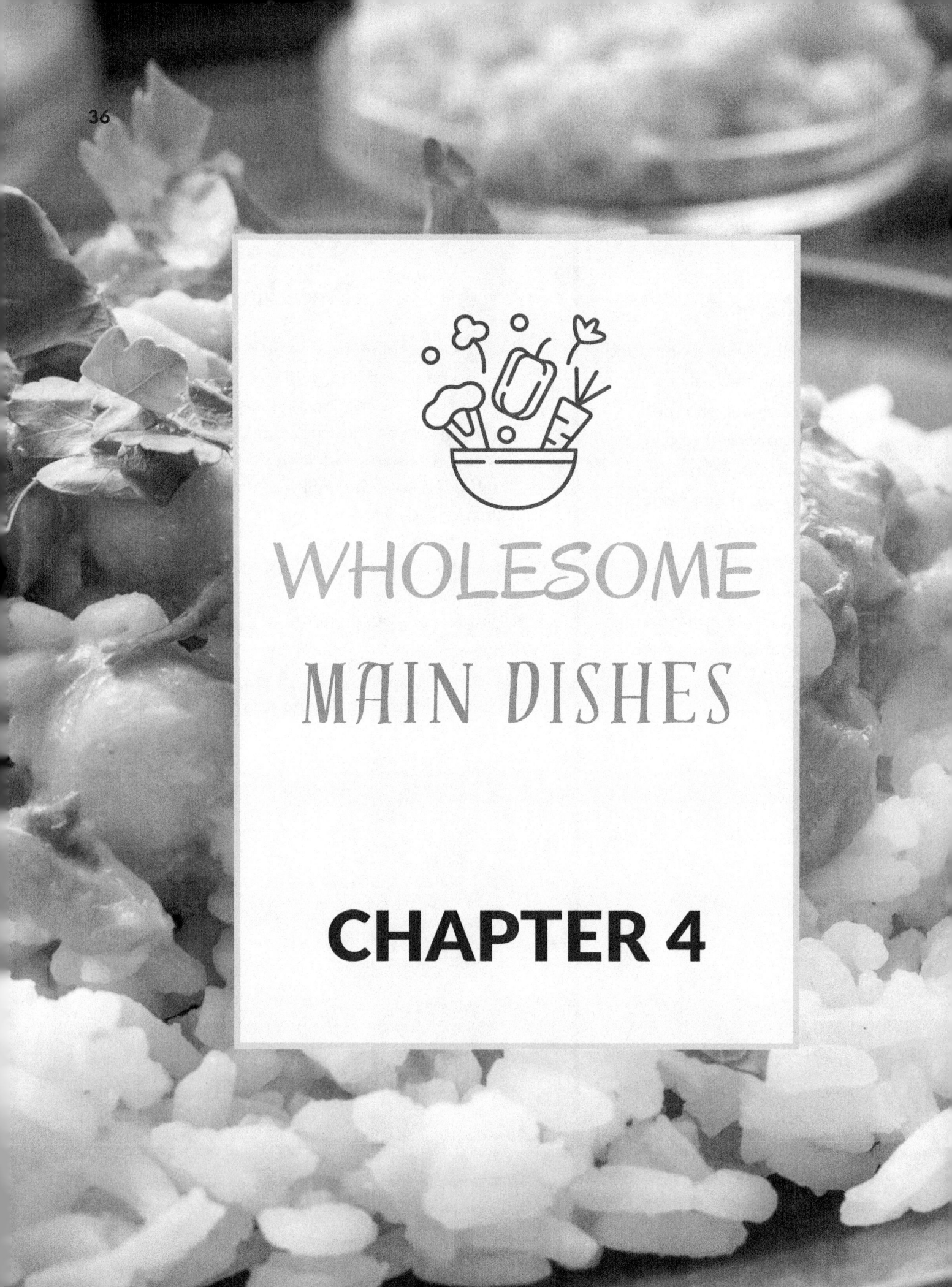

WHOLESOME MAIN DISHES

CHAPTER 4

Lentil and Vegetable Curry

Servings: 2   Prep Time: 10 mins   Cook Time: 25 mins   Total Time: 35 mins

Ingredients

1 tablespoon olive oil

1 small onion, diced

2 cloves garlic, minced

1 teaspoon ground cumin

1 teaspoon ground coriander

1/2 teaspoon ground turmeric

1/4 teaspoon ground ginger

1/4 teaspoon ground cinnamon

1 cup diced tomatoes (fresh or canned)

1 cup vegetable broth

1/2 cup dried green lentils, rinsed and drained

1 cup chopped mixed vegetables (such as carrots, bell peppers, zucchini)

1/2 cup coconut milk

Fresh cilantro leaves, for garnish

Procedures

1. Heat olive oil in a large skillet over medium heat. Add diced onion and cook until translucent, about 3-4 minutes.
2. Add minced garlic, ground cumin, ground coriander, ground turmeric, ground ginger, and ground cinnamon to the skillet. Cook for 1-2 minutes, stirring constantly, until fragrant.
3. Stir in diced tomatoes, vegetable broth, and dried green lentils. Bring to a simmer, then reduce heat to low and cover. Let the mixture cook for 15-20 minutes, or until lentils are tender.
4. Add chopped mixed vegetables to the skillet and cook for an additional 5-7 minutes, or until vegetables are tender.
5. Stir in coconut milk and cook for another 2-3 minutes, until heated through.
6. Serve the lentil and vegetable curry hot, garnished with fresh cilantro leaves.

Nutritional Value (per serving): Calories: 320 Kcal, Carbohydrates: 40 g, Proteins: 13 g, Fats: 14 g, Sodium: 150 mg, Potassium: 700 mg, Fiber: 12 g, Sugar: 7 g

Eggplant Parmesan with Whole Wheat Pasta

Servings: 2   Prep Time: 15 mins   Cook Time: 40 mins   Total Time: 55 mins

Ingredients

1 medium eggplant, sliced into rounds

1 cup whole wheat pasta

1 cup marinara sauce (no added sugar)

1/2 cup grated Parmesan cheese (or vegan alternative)

1 tablespoon olive oil

1 teaspoon dried oregano

1 teaspoon dried basil

1/2 teaspoon garlic powder

1/4 teaspoon black pepper

Cooking spray

Procedures

1. Preheat your oven to 375°F (190°C). Lightly grease a baking sheet with cooking spray.
2. Place the eggplant slices on the prepared baking sheet. Drizzle olive oil over the slices and sprinkle with dried oregano, basil, garlic powder, and black pepper.
3. Bake the eggplant slices in the preheated oven for 25-30 minutes, or until tender and lightly golden brown.
4. While the eggplant is baking, cook the whole wheat pasta according to the package instructions. Drain and set aside.
5. Once the eggplant is done, remove it from the oven and increase the oven temperature to 400°F (200°C).
6. In a small baking dish, spread a thin layer of marinara sauce. Place half of the baked eggplant slices on top of the sauce.
7. Top the eggplant slices with another layer of marinara sauce and sprinkle with half of the grated Parmesan cheese.
8. Repeat the layers with the remaining eggplant slices, marinara sauce, and Parmesan cheese.
9. Bake the assembled dish in the preheated oven for 10-15 minutes, or until the cheese is melted and bubbly.
10. Serve the Eggplant Parmesan hot over cooked whole wheat pasta.

Nutritional Value (per serving): Calories: 380 Kcal, Carbohydrates: 54 g, Proteins: 15 g, Fats: 12 g, Sodium:

Black Bean and Sweet Potato Enchiladas

Servings: 2 Prep Time: 15 mins   Cook Time: 40 mins   Total Time: 55 mins

Ingredients

1 medium sweet potato, peeled and diced

1 cup cooked black beans

1/2 cup diced onion

1 clove garlic, minced

1/2 teaspoon ground cumin

1/2 teaspoon paprika

1/4 teaspoon chili powder

1/4 teaspoon ground coriander

1/4 teaspoon dried oregano

1/4 teaspoon black pepper

1/4 cup chopped fresh cilantro

1/2 cup tomato sauce

4 small corn tortillas

1/2 cup shredded lettuce

1/4 cup diced tomatoes

1/4 cup diced avocado

Lime wedges, for serving

Procedures

1. Preheat the oven to 375°F (190°C).
2. In a skillet over medium heat, add the diced sweet potato and cook until tender, about 10 minutes.
3. Add the diced onion and minced garlic to the skillet and cook for an additional 2-3 minutes until softened.
4. Stir in the cooked black beans, ground cumin, paprika, chili powder, ground coriander, dried oregano, black pepper, and half of the chopped cilantro. Cook for another 2 minutes until well combined.
5. Spread a thin layer of tomato sauce on the bottom of a baking dish.
6. Spoon the sweet potato and black bean mixture evenly onto each corn tortilla, then roll them up tightly and place them seam side down in the baking dish.
7. Pour the remaining tomato sauce over the enchiladas, spreading it evenly.
8. Bake in the preheated oven for 20-25 minutes, until the enchiladas are heated through and the sauce is bubbly.
9. Remove from the oven and garnish with the remaining chopped cilantro.
10. Serve the enchiladas with shredded lettuce, diced tomatoes, diced avocado, and lime wedges on the side.

Nutritional Value (per serving): Calories: 375 Kcal, Carbohydrates: 63 g, Proteins: 11 g, Fats: 9 g, Sodium: 210 mg, Potassium: 960 mg, Fiber: 15 g, Sugar: 8 g

Veggie Stir-Fry with Cashews

Servings: 2   Prep Time: 10 mins   Cook Time: 15 mins   Total Time: 25 mins

Ingredients

1 tablespoon olive oil

2 cloves garlic, minced

1 small onion, thinly sliced

1 bell pepper, thinly sliced

1 cup broccoli florets

1 cup sliced carrots

1 cup sliced mushrooms

1/4 cup cashews

1 teaspoon ginger, grated

1/2 teaspoon turmeric powder

1/2 teaspoon paprika

1/2 teaspoon cumin

Freshly ground black pepper, to taste

Fresh herbs (such as cilantro or parsley), for garnish

Procedures

1. In a large skillet or wok, heat olive oil over medium heat. Add minced garlic and grated ginger, and sauté for 1-2 minutes until fragrant.
2. Add sliced onion to the skillet and cook for 2-3 minutes until translucent.
3. Add broccoli florets, sliced carrots, and bell pepper to the skillet. Cook for 5-6 minutes until vegetables are tender-crisp.
4. Stir in sliced mushrooms and cashews, and cook for an additional 2-3 minutes until mushrooms are cooked through.
5. Sprinkle turmeric powder, paprika, cumin, and freshly ground black pepper over the vegetables, and toss to coat evenly.
6. Cook for another 1-2 minutes to allow the flavors to meld together.
7. Remove from heat and transfer the veggie stir-fry to serving plates.
8. Garnish with fresh herbs, such as cilantro or parsley, for an extra burst of flavor.
9. Serve hot and enjoy.

Lentil Shepherd's Pie with Mashed Cauliflower Topping

Servings: 2 Prep Time: 15 mins   Cook Time: 35 mins   Total Time: 50 mins

Ingredients

For the Lentil Filling:
1 cup dry green or brown lentils, rinsed

2 cups vegetable broth

1 tablespoon olive oil

1 onion, diced

2 cloves garlic, minced

1 carrot, diced

1 celery stalk, diced

1 teaspoon dried thyme

1 teaspoon dried rosemary

1 teaspoon paprika

1 tablespoon tomato paste

1 tablespoon low-sodium soy sauce or tamari

1 tablespoon cornstarch mixed with 2 tablespoons water (optional, for thickening)

Freshly ground black pepper, to taste

For the Mashed Cauliflower Topping:
1 small head cauliflower, chopped into florets

2 cloves garlic, minced

2 tablespoons unsweetened almond milk or vegetable broth

1 tablespoon nutritional yeast

1 teaspoon dried parsley

Freshly ground black pepper, to taste

Procedures

1. Preheat the oven to 400°F (200°C).
2. In a medium saucepan, combine the lentils and vegetable broth. Bring to a boil, then reduce heat, cover, and simmer for about 20-25 minutes, or until the lentils are tender and most of the liquid is absorbed.
3. Meanwhile, heat the olive oil in a large skillet over medium heat. Add the diced onion, garlic, carrot, and celery. Sauté for 5-7 minutes, or until the vegetables are softened.
4. Add the thyme, rosemary, paprika, tomato paste, and soy sauce to the skillet. Stir to combine and cook for another 2 minutes.
5. If desired, stir in the cornstarch mixture to thicken the filling. Then, add the cooked lentils to the skillet and mix well. Season with black pepper to taste. Remove from heat and set aside.
6. While the lentil filling is cooking, steam the cauliflower florets until tender, about 10-12 minutes. Drain well.
7. Transfer the steamed cauliflower to a food processor. Add the minced garlic, almond milk or vegetable broth, nutritional yeast, dried parsley, and black pepper. Blend until smooth and creamy.
8. In a small baking dish or individual ramekins, spoon the lentil filling evenly. Top with the mashed cauliflower, spreading it out evenly over the lentils.
9. Place the dish(es) in the preheated oven and bake for 15-20 minutes, or until the top is lightly golden.
10. Remove from the oven and let cool for a few minutes before serving.

Nutritional Value (per serving): Calories: 320 Kcal, Carbohydrates: 52 g, Proteins: 20 g, Fats: 5 g, Sodium: 130 mg, Potassium: 1160 mg, Fiber: 20 g, Sugar: 8 g

Vegetable Paella with Saffron Rice

Servings: 2 Prep Time: 15 mins   Cook Time: 30 mins   Total Time: 45 mins

Ingredients

1 cup brown rice

2 cups vegetable broth (low sodium)

1/4 teaspoon saffron threads

1 tablespoon olive oil

1 small onion, diced

2 cloves garlic, minced

1 red bell pepper, diced

1 yellow bell pepper, diced

1 zucchini, diced

1 cup cherry tomatoes, halved

1/2 cup green peas

1 teaspoon smoked paprika

1/2 teaspoon ground turmeric

1/2 teaspoon dried thyme

1/2 teaspoon dried oregano

1/4 teaspoon black pepper

1/4 cup chopped fresh parsley

Lemon wedges, for serving

Procedures

1. In a small bowl, combine the saffron threads with 2 tablespoons of warm water. Let it sit and steep while you prepare the rest of the ingredients.
2. Rinse the brown rice under cold water until the water runs clear. In a medium saucepan, bring the vegetable broth to a boil. Add the rinsed rice and saffron-infused water to the saucepan. Reduce the heat to low, cover, and simmer for about 20-25 minutes, or until the rice is cooked and the liquid is absorbed.
3. While the rice is cooking, heat the olive oil in a large skillet over medium heat. Add the diced onion and cook until softened, about 3-4 minutes. Add the minced garlic and cook for another minute until fragrant.
4. Add the diced bell peppers, zucchini, cherry tomatoes, and green peas to the skillet. Cook for 5-6 minutes, stirring occasionally, until the vegetables are tender but still slightly crisp.
5. Stir in the smoked paprika, ground turmeric, dried thyme, dried oregano, and black pepper. Cook for another minute to allow the flavors to meld.
6. Once the rice is cooked, fluff it with a fork and add it to the skillet with the cooked vegetables. Gently toss everything together until well combined.
7. Remove the skillet from the heat and sprinkle the chopped fresh parsley over the vegetable paella. Serve warm with lemon wedges on the side.

Nutritional Value (per serving): Calories: 345 Kcal, Carbohydrates: 63 g, Proteins: 8 g, Fats: 7 g, Sodium: 127 mg, Potassium: 719 mg, Fiber: 9 g, Sugar: 8 g

Servings: 2 Prep Time: 15 mins   Cook Time: 30 mins   Total Time: 45 mins

Ingredients

2 medium sweet potatoes, peeled and diced

2 cups kale, chopped

1 tablespoon olive oil

1 teaspoon paprika

1/2 teaspoon garlic powder

1/2 teaspoon onion powder

1/4 teaspoon black pepper

4 large eggs

Chopped fresh parsley or cilantro, for garnish

Procedures

1. Heat olive oil in a large skillet over medium heat.
2. Add diced sweet potatoes to the skillet and cook for about 8-10 minutes, or until they start to soften, stirring occasionally.
3. Add chopped kale to the skillet along with paprika, garlic powder, onion powder, and black pepper. Stir well to combine.
4. Continue cooking for another 5-7 minutes, or until the sweet potatoes are tender and the kale is wilted.
5. While the hash is cooking, poach the eggs. Bring a pot of water to a gentle simmer, then carefully crack the eggs into the water and poach for 3-4 minutes, until the whites are set but the yolks are still runny.
6. Once the sweet potato and kale hash is cooked, divide it evenly between two plates.
7. Top each serving with two poached eggs.
8. Garnish with chopped fresh parsley or cilantro.
9. Serve immediately and enjoy!

Nutritional Value (per serving): Calories: 287 kcal, Carbohydrates: 31 g, Proteins: 14 g, Fats: 14 g, Sodium:

NOURISHING SIDE DISHES

CHAPTER 5

Grilled asparagus with lemon zest

Servings: 2 Prep Time: 5 mins   Cook Time: 10 mins   Total Time: 15 mins

Ingredients

1 bunch of asparagus spears, trimmed

1 tablespoon olive oil

1 teaspoon dried thyme

1 teaspoon dried rosemary

Zest of 1 lemon

Freshly ground black pepper, to taste

Procedures

1. Preheat your grill to medium-high heat.
2. In a small bowl, mix together olive oil, dried thyme, dried rosemary, and lemon zest.
3. Place the trimmed asparagus spears in a shallow dish and coat them with the olive oil mixture, ensuring they are evenly coated.
4. Place the asparagus spears directly on the grill and cook for about 5-7 minutes, turning occasionally, until they are tender and slightly charred.
5. Remove the grilled asparagus from the grill and transfer them to a serving plate.
6. Sprinkle freshly ground black pepper over the grilled asparagus before serving.
7. Enjoy your delicious and nutritious grilled asparagus with lemon zest!

Nutritional Value (per serving): Calories: 78 Kcal, Carbohydrates: 5 g, Proteins: 3 g, Fats: 6 g, Sodium: 2 mg, Potassium: 300 mg, Fiber: 3 g, Sugar: 2 g

Baked sweet potato fries with paprika

Servings: 2   Prep Time: 10 mins   Cook Time: 25 mins   Total Time: 35 mins

Ingredients

2 medium sweet potatoes, scrubbed
and cut into thin fries
1 tablespoon olive oil
1 teaspoon paprika
1/2 teaspoon garlic powder
1/2 teaspoon onion powder
1/2 teaspoon dried thyme
1/2 teaspoon dried rosemary
1/4 teaspoon black pepper
Cooking spray (optional)

Procedures

1. Preheat your oven to 425°F (220°C). Line a baking sheet with parchment paper or lightly grease it with cooking spray.
2. In a large bowl, toss the sweet potato fries with olive oil until evenly coated.
3. In a small bowl, mix together the paprika, garlic powder, onion powder, dried thyme, dried rosemary, and black pepper.
4. Sprinkle the seasoning mixture over the sweet potato fries and toss until the fries are evenly coated with the seasoning.
5. Arrange the seasoned sweet potato fries in a single layer on the prepared baking sheet, making sure they're not overcrowded.
6. Bake in the preheated oven for 20-25 minutes, flipping halfway through, until the fries are crispy and golden brown.
7. Once done, remove from the oven and let cool slightly before serving.

Nutritional Value (per serving): Calories: 160 Kcal, Carbohydrates: 28 g, Proteins: 2 g, Fats: 5 g, Sodium: 36 mg, Potassium: 389 mg, Fiber: 5 g, Sugar: 6 g

Roasted carrots with honey and thyme

Servings: 2 Prep Time: 10 mins   Cook Time: 25 mins   Total Time: 35 mins

Ingredients

4 medium-sized carrots, peeled and
sliced into sticks
1 tablespoon olive oil
1 tablespoon honey
1 teaspoon fresh thyme leaves
1/2 teaspoon ground black pepper
1/2 teaspoon garlic powder

Procedures

1. Preheat your oven to 400°F (200°C) and line a baking sheet with parchment paper.
2. In a small bowl, mix together the olive oil, honey, fresh thyme leaves, black pepper, and garlic powder until well combined.
3. Place the sliced carrots on the prepared baking sheet and drizzle the honey and herb mixture over them. Toss gently to coat the carrots evenly.
4. Spread the carrots out in a single layer on the baking sheet, ensuring they are not overcrowded.
5. Roast in the preheated oven for about 25 minutes or until the carrots are tender and caramelized, stirring halfway through the cooking time.
6. Once roasted, remove the carrots from the oven and serve hot as a delicious side dish to your favorite main course.

Nutritional Value (per serving): Calories: 95 Kcal, Carbohydrates: 15 g, Proteins: 1 g, Fats: 4 g, Sodium: 40 mg, Potassium: 368 mg, Fiber: 3 g, Sugar: 9 g

Zucchini noodles with pesto sauce

Servings: 2 Prep Time: 10 mins Cook Time: 10 mins Total Time: 20 mins

Ingredients

2 medium zucchinis

1 cup fresh basil leaves

2 tablespoons pine nuts

2 cloves garlic, minced

2 tablespoons nutritional yeast

2 tablespoons olive oil

1 tablespoon lemon juice

1 tablespoon water

Black pepper, to taste

Crushed red pepper flakes, to taste

Procedures

1. Spiralize the zucchinis into noodles using a spiralizer or a vegetable peeler. Set aside.
2. In a food processor or blender, combine the basil leaves, pine nuts, minced garlic, nutritional yeast, olive oil, lemon juice, and water. Blend until smooth and creamy, adding more water if needed to reach your desired consistency.
3. Heat a non-stick skillet over medium heat. Add the zucchini noodles and cook for 3-4 minutes, or until just tender.
4. Once the zucchini noodles are cooked, transfer them to a serving plate. Top with the prepared pesto sauce.
5. Garnish with black pepper and crushed red pepper flakes, to taste.
6. Serve immediately and enjoy!

Nutritional Value (per serving): Calories: 180 Kcal, Carbohydrates: 10 g, Proteins: 5 g, Fats: 14 g, Sodium: 5 mg, Potassium: 420 mg, Fiber: 3 g, Sugar: 4 g

Corn and black bean salsa with lime and cilantro

Servings: 2   Prep Time: 10 mins   Cook Time: 0 min   Total Time: 10 mins

Ingredients

1 cup cooked black beans, drained and rinsed

1 cup corn kernels (fresh, frozen, or canned)

1 small red bell pepper, diced

1 small jalapeno pepper, seeds removed and finely chopped

2 tablespoons fresh cilantro, chopped

1 tablespoon lime juice

1 teaspoon ground cumin

1/2 teaspoon smoked paprika

1/4 teaspoon garlic powder

Freshly ground black pepper, to taste

Procedures

1. In a mixing bowl, combine the black beans, corn, diced red bell pepper, chopped jalapeno pepper, and chopped cilantro.
2. In a small bowl, whisk together the lime juice, ground cumin, smoked paprika, garlic powder, and black pepper.
3. Pour the lime juice mixture over the bean and corn mixture, and toss until well combined and evenly coated.
4. Taste and adjust seasoning if necessary.
5. Serve immediately or refrigerate for at least 30 minutes to allow the flavors to meld together.

Nutritional Value (per serving): Calories: 180 Kcal, Carbohydrates: 35 g, Proteins: 9 g, Fats: 1 g, Sodium: 15 mg, Potassium: 540 mg, Fiber: 9 g, Sugar: 4 g

Cabbage slaw with apple cider vinegar dressing

Servings: 2   Prep Time: 10 mins   Cook Time: 0 min   Total Time: 10 mins

Ingredients

2 cups shredded cabbage

1 medium carrot, grated

1/4 cup chopped fresh parsley

1 tablespoon apple cider vinegar

1 tablespoon extra virgin olive oil

1 teaspoon dijon mustard

1/2 teaspoon black pepper

1/2 teaspoon dried oregano

1/2 teaspoon dried thyme

Procedures

1. In a large mixing bowl, combine the shredded cabbage, grated carrot, and chopped parsley.
2. In a small bowl, whisk together the apple cider vinegar, olive oil, dijon mustard, black pepper, dried oregano, and dried thyme until well combined.
3. Pour the dressing over the cabbage mixture and toss until everything is evenly coated.
4. Serve immediately or refrigerate for 30 minutes to allow the flavors to meld together.

Nutritional Value (per serving): Calories: 85 Kcal, Carbohydrates: 7 g, Proteins: 1 g, Fats: 6 g, Sodium: 12 mg, Potassium: 189 mg, Fiber: 3 g, Sugar: 3 g

Servings: 2 Prep Time: 10 mins   Cook Time: 25 mins   Total Time: 35 mins

Ingredients

For the Spicy Roasted Cauliflower:

1 small head cauliflower, cut into florets

2 tablespoons olive oil

1 teaspoon paprika

1/2 teaspoon cumin

1/2 teaspoon garlic powder

1/4 teaspoon chili powder

Freshly ground black pepper, to taste

For the Tahini Dipping Sauce:

2 tablespoons tahini

1 tablespoon lemon juice

1 clove garlic, minced

2 tablespoons water

Pinch of cayenne pepper (optional)

Fresh parsley, chopped, for garnish

Procedures

1. Preheat your oven to 400°F (200°C) and line a baking sheet with parchment paper.
2. In a large bowl, toss the cauliflower florets with olive oil until evenly coated.
3. In a small bowl, mix together the paprika, cumin, garlic powder, chili powder, and black pepper.
4. Sprinkle the spice mixture over the cauliflower florets and toss until they are well coated.
5. Spread the cauliflower in a single layer on the prepared baking sheet.
6. Roast in the preheated oven for 20-25 minutes, or until the cauliflower is tender and golden brown, stirring halfway through.
7. While the cauliflower is roasting, prepare the tahini dipping sauce. In a small bowl, whisk together the tahini, lemon juice, minced garlic, water, and cayenne pepper (if using) until smooth and creamy. Add more water if needed to achieve your desired consistency.
8. Once the cauliflower is done, remove it from the oven and transfer to a serving plate.
9. Garnish with chopped fresh parsley and serve hot with the tahini dipping sauce on the side.

Nutritional Value (per serving): Calories: 185 Kcal, Carbohydrates: 12 g, Proteins: 5 g, Fats: 14 g, Sodium: 34

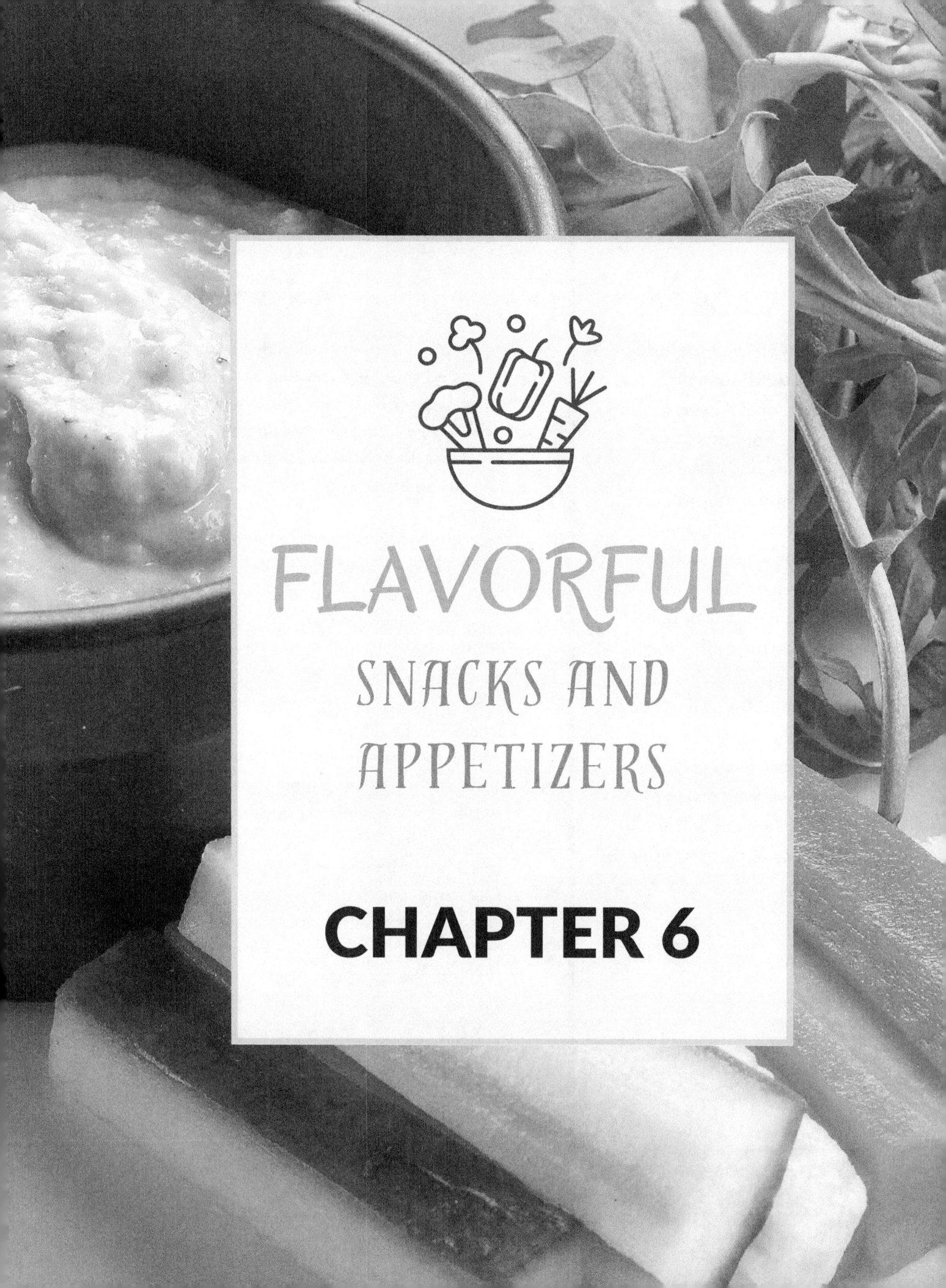

FLAVORFUL
SNACKS AND APPETIZERS

CHAPTER 6

Hummus with Crudites

Servings: 2   Prep Time: 10 mins   Cook Time: 0 min   Total Time: 10 mins

Ingredients

1 can (15 ounces) chickpeas, drained and rinsed

2 tablespoons tahini

2 tablespoons lemon juice

2 cloves garlic, minced

1/2 teaspoon ground cumin

1/4 teaspoon paprika

1/4 teaspoon black pepper

2 tablespoons water

Assorted vegetables (carrot sticks, cucumber slices, bell pepper strips) for serving

Procedures

1. In a food processor, combine the chickpeas, tahini, lemon juice, minced garlic, ground cumin, paprika, and black pepper.
2. Blend the mixture until smooth and creamy, scraping down the sides of the processor as needed.
3. If the hummus is too thick, add water, one tablespoon at a time, until desired consistency is reached.
4. Transfer the hummus to a serving bowl and garnish with a sprinkle of paprika and a drizzle of olive oil, if desired.
5. Serve the hummus with assorted crudites such as carrot sticks, cucumber slices, and bell pepper strips.

Nutritional Value (per serving): Calories: 160 Kcal, Carbohydrates: 20 g, Proteins: 7 g, Fats: 7 g, Sodium: 120 mg, Potassium: 220 mg, Fiber: 6 g, Sugar: 1 g

Spinach and Artichoke Dip with Whole Wheat Pita Chips

Servings: 2   Prep Time: 10 mins   Cook Time: 20 mins   Total Time: 30 mins

Ingredients

For the Spinach and Artichoke Dip:

1 cup chopped spinach

1/2 cup canned artichoke hearts, drained and chopped

1/2 cup plain Greek yogurt (non-fat)

2 tablespoons nutritional yeast

1 tablespoon olive oil

1 teaspoon minced garlic

1/2 teaspoon dried basil

1/2 teaspoon dried oregano

1/4 teaspoon black pepper

For the Whole Wheat Pita Chips:

2 whole wheat pita bread rounds

1 teaspoon olive oil

1/4 teaspoon dried thyme

1/4 teaspoon dried rosemary

1/4 teaspoon dried parsley

Procedures

1. Preheat the oven to 375°F (190°C).
2. In a mixing bowl, combine chopped spinach, chopped artichoke hearts, Greek yogurt, nutritional yeast, olive oil, minced garlic, dried basil, dried oregano, and black pepper. Mix well until all ingredients are evenly incorporated.
3. Spread the spinach and artichoke mixture evenly into a small baking dish.
4. Cut the whole wheat pita bread rounds into triangles. Place them on a baking sheet lined with parchment paper.
5. In a small bowl, combine olive oil, dried thyme, dried rosemary, and dried parsley. Brush the mixture onto both sides of the pita triangles.
6. Place the baking dish with the spinach and artichoke mixture and the baking sheet with the pita triangles into the preheated oven.
7. Bake for about 15-20 minutes, or until the dip is heated through and bubbly, and the pita chips are golden and crispy.
8. Remove from the oven and let cool for a few minutes before serving.

Nutritional Value (per serving): Calories: 220 Kcal, Carbohydrates: 28 g, Proteins: 12 g, Fats: 8 g, Sodium: 150 mg, Potassium: 350 mg, Fiber: 6 g, Sugar: 2 g

Baked Sweet Potato Fries with Chipotle Aioli

Servings: 2 Prep Time: 10 mins   Cook Time: 25 mins   Total Time: 35 mins

Ingredients

For the Sweet Potato Fries:

2 medium sweet potatoes, washed and cut into thin strips

1 tablespoon olive oil

1 teaspoon paprika

1/2 teaspoon garlic powder

1/2 teaspoon onion powder

1/4 teaspoon black pepper

For the Chipotle Aioli:

1/4 cup plain Greek yogurt

1 tablespoon lemon juice

1 clove garlic, minced

1 teaspoon chipotle powder

1/4 teaspoon smoked paprika

1/4 teaspoon cumin

Fresh parsley, for garnish

Procedures

1. Preheat your oven to 425°F (220°C) and line a baking sheet with parchment paper.
2. In a large bowl, toss the sweet potato strips with olive oil, paprika, garlic powder, onion powder, and black pepper until evenly coated.
3. Arrange the seasoned sweet potato strips on the prepared baking sheet in a single layer, making sure they're not overcrowded.
4. Bake in the preheated oven for 20-25 minutes, flipping halfway through, until the fries are golden brown and crispy.
5. While the fries are baking, prepare the chipotle aioli. In a small bowl, whisk together Greek yogurt, lemon juice, minced garlic, chipotle powder, smoked paprika, and cumin until well combined.
6. Once the sweet potato fries are done, remove them from the oven and let them cool slightly.
7. Serve the baked sweet potato fries hot, garnished with fresh parsley, alongside the chipotle aioli for dipping.

Spicy Roasted Cauliflower Bites

Servings: 2   Prep Time: 10 mins   Cook Time: 25 mins   Total Time: 35 mins

Ingredients

1 small head cauliflower, cut into florets

2 tablespoons olive oil

1 teaspoon paprika

1/2 teaspoon cumin

1/4 teaspoon garlic powder

1/4 teaspoon onion powder

1/4 teaspoon chili powder

1/4 teaspoon black pepper

Fresh parsley, chopped, for garnish

Procedures

1. Preheat your oven to 400°F (200°C) and line a baking sheet with parchment paper.
2. In a large bowl, toss the cauliflower florets with olive oil until evenly coated.
3. In a small bowl, mix together paprika, cumin, garlic powder, onion powder, chili powder, and black pepper.
4. Sprinkle the spice mixture over the cauliflower florets and toss until well combined.
5. Spread the seasoned cauliflower in a single layer on the prepared baking sheet.
6. Roast in the preheated oven for 20-25 minutes, or until the cauliflower is tender and golden brown, stirring halfway through.
7. Once roasted, remove from the oven and garnish with chopped fresh parsley.
8. Serve hot as a delicious and nutritious side dish.

Nutritional Value (per serving): Calories: 120 Kcal, Carbohydrates: 8 g, Proteins: 3 g, Fats: 9 g, Sodium: 28 mg, Potassium: 430 mg, Fiber: 3 g, Sugar: 3 g

Cucumber Cups filled with Tzatziki and Diced Vegetables

Servings: 2   Prep Time: 10 mins   Cook Time: 25 mins   Total Time: 35 mins

Ingredients

1 large cucumber

1/2 cup diced tomatoes

1/4 cup diced red onion

1/4 cup diced bell pepper (any color)

1/4 cup diced cucumber (from the removed flesh)

1/4 cup plain Greek yogurt (fat-free)

1/4 cup grated cucumber (from the removed flesh)

1 clove garlic, minced

1 tablespoon chopped fresh dill

1 tablespoon chopped fresh parsley

1 tablespoon lemon juice

Black pepper, to taste

Paprika, for garnish

Procedures

1. Begin by preparing the cucumber cups. Cut the cucumber into thick slices, about 2 inches wide. Use a melon baller or spoon to hollow out the center of each cucumber slice, creating a cup-like shape. Reserve the removed flesh for later use.
2. In a small bowl, combine the diced tomatoes, red onion, bell pepper, and diced cucumber. Set aside.
3. In another bowl, mix the plain Greek yogurt, grated cucumber, minced garlic, chopped dill, chopped parsley, lemon juice, and black pepper. Stir until well combined to create the tzatziki sauce.
4. Fill each cucumber cup with a spoonful of the tzatziki sauce, then top with the diced vegetable mixture.
5. Garnish the filled cucumber cups with a sprinkle of paprika for added flavor and visual appeal.
6. Serve immediately and enjoy.

Nutritional Value (per serving): Calories: 70 Kcal, Carbohydrates: 10 g, Proteins: 6 g, Fats: 1 g, Sodium: 30 mg, Potassium: 380 mg, Fiber: 2 g, Sugar: 5 g

Mango Salsa with Baked Tortilla Chips

Servings: 2   Prep Time: 10 mins   Cook Time: 10 mins   Total Time: 20 mins

Ingredients

For Mango Salsa:

1 ripe mango, diced

1/4 cup red onion, finely chopped

1/4 cup fresh cilantro, chopped

1 small jalapeño pepper, seeded and minced

1 tablespoon lime juice

1/2 teaspoon ground cumin

1/4 teaspoon paprika

1/4 teaspoon black pepper

For Baked Tortilla Chips:

2 whole grain tortillas

Cooking spray

Procedures

1. Preheat your oven to 350°F (175°C).
2. In a mixing bowl, combine diced mango, chopped red onion, minced jalapeño pepper, and chopped cilantro.
3. Add lime juice, ground cumin, paprika, and black pepper to the mango mixture. Stir until well combined. Set aside.
4. Cut each whole grain tortilla into wedges or desired chip size.
5. Arrange the tortilla wedges on a baking sheet lined with parchment paper.
6. Lightly spray the tortilla wedges with cooking spray.
7. Bake in the preheated oven for 8-10 minutes, or until the tortilla chips are crispy and golden brown.
8. Remove the baked tortilla chips from the oven and let them cool slightly.
9. Serve the mango salsa alongside the baked tortilla chips.

Nutritional Value (per serving): Calories: 130 Kcal, Carbohydrates: 29 g, Proteins: 3 g, Fats: 1 g, Sodium: 3 mg, Potassium: 361 mg, Fiber: 5 g, Sugar: 14 g

Roasted Red Pepper and White Bean Dip with Whole Grain Pita Bread

Servings: 2 Prep Time: 10 mins   Cook Time: 25 mins   Total Time: 35 mins

Ingredients

1 large red bell pepper
1 can (15 oz) white beans, drained and rinsed
1 tablespoon olive oil
1 tablespoon lemon juice
1 clove garlic, minced
1 teaspoon dried oregano
1/2 teaspoon smoked paprika
1/4 teaspoon black pepper
Whole grain pita bread, for serving

Procedures

1. Preheat the oven to 425°F (220°C). Line a baking sheet with parchment paper.
2. Cut the red bell pepper in half, remove the seeds, and place it cut side down on the prepared baking sheet.
3. Roast the pepper in the preheated oven for 20-25 minutes, until the skin is blistered and charred.
4. Remove the pepper from the oven and let it cool for a few minutes. Then, peel off the skin and discard.
5. In a food processor, combine the roasted red pepper, white beans, olive oil, lemon juice, minced garlic, dried oregano, smoked paprika, and black pepper.
6. Blend until smooth and creamy, scraping down the sides of the food processor as needed.
7. Transfer the dip to a serving bowl and garnish with a sprinkle of oregano or paprika, if desired.
8. Serve the roasted red pepper and white bean dip with whole grain pita bread for dipping.

Nutritional Value (per serving): Calories: 180 Kcal, Carbohydrates: 25 g, Proteins: 8 g, Fats: 6 g, Sodium: 10 mg, Potassium: 370 mg, Fiber: 6 g, Sugar: 2 g

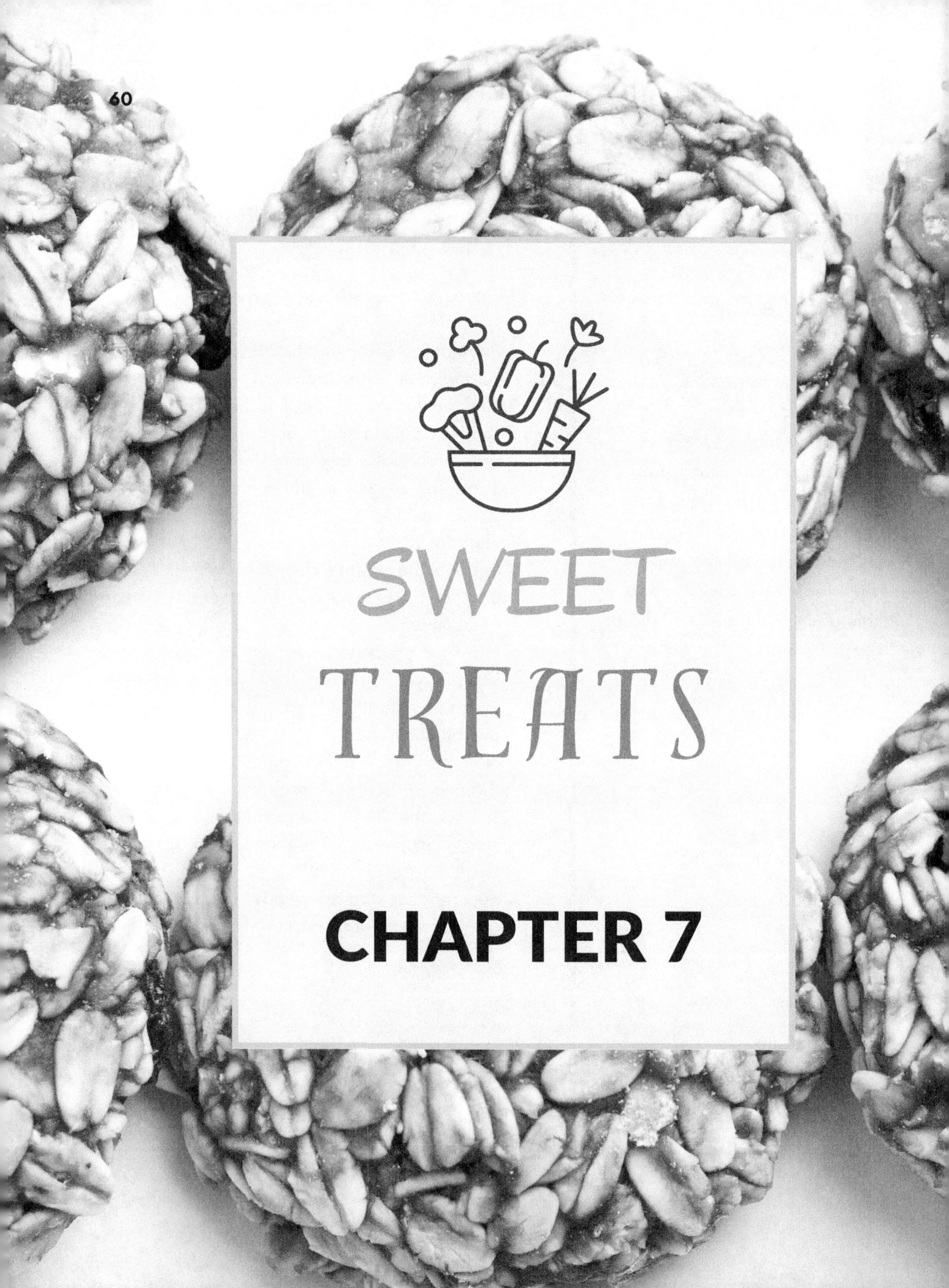

SWEET
TREATS

CHAPTER 7

Banana-Oat Cookies

Servings: 2   Prep Time: 10 mins   Cook Time: 15 mins   Total Time: 25 mins

Ingredients

1 ripe banana, mashed

1/2 cup rolled oats

1 tablespoon almond butter

1 tablespoon maple syrup

1/2 teaspoon cinnamon

1/4 teaspoon nutmeg

1/4 teaspoon vanilla extract

Procedures

1. Preheat your oven to 350°F (175°C) and line a baking sheet with parchment paper.
2. In a mixing bowl, combine the mashed banana, rolled oats, almond butter, maple syrup, cinnamon, nutmeg, and vanilla extract. Mix well until all ingredients are evenly combined.
3. Using a spoon, scoop the cookie dough onto the prepared baking sheet, shaping them into cookie shapes.
4. Bake in the preheated oven for 12-15 minutes, or until the cookies are golden brown and set.
5. Once baked, remove the cookies from the oven and let them cool on the baking sheet for a few minutes before transferring them to a wire rack to cool completely.

Nutritional Value (per serving): Calories: 160 Kcal, Carbohydrates: 30 g, Proteins: 3 g, Fats: 4 g, Sodium: 2 mg, Potassium: 316 mg, Fiber: 4 g, Sugar: 12 g

Mango Coconut Nice Cream

Servings: 2 Prep Time: 10 mins Cook Time: 0 min Total Time: 4 hours + 10 mins

Ingredients

2 ripe mangoes, peeled and diced

1/2 cup canned coconut milk

1 tablespoon maple syrup or honey (optional, adjust to taste)

1 teaspoon vanilla extract

1/2 teaspoon ground cinnamon

1/4 teaspoon ground ginger

Fresh mint leaves, for garnish

Procedures

1. In a blender or food processor, combine the diced mangoes, canned coconut milk, maple syrup or honey (if using), vanilla extract, ground cinnamon, and ground ginger.
2. Blend until smooth and creamy, scraping down the sides of the blender as needed to ensure all ingredients are well incorporated.
3. Once the mixture is smooth, taste and adjust sweetness if necessary by adding more maple syrup or honey.
4. Transfer the mixture to a shallow container and freeze for at least 4 hours or until firm.
5. When ready to serve, allow the nice cream to sit at room temperature for a few minutes to soften slightly. Then, scoop into bowls, garnish with fresh mint leaves, and enjoy!

Nutritional Value (per serving): Calories: 180 Kcal, Carbohydrates: 35 g, Proteins: 2 g, Fats: 6 g, Sodium: 10 mg, Potassium: 460 mg, Fiber: 4 g, Sugar: 30 g

Mixed Berry Crisp with Oat Topping

Servings: 2 Prep Time: 10 mins Cook Time: 25 mins   Total Time: 35 mins

Ingredients

2 cups mixed berries (such as strawberries, blueberries, raspberries)

2 tablespoons maple syrup

1 tablespoon lemon juice

1/2 teaspoon ground cinnamon

1/4 teaspoon ground nutmeg

1/2 cup old-fashioned oats

1/4 cup almond flour

2 tablespoons chopped nuts (such as almonds or walnuts)

2 tablespoons coconut oil, melted

1 tablespoon maple syrup

1/2 teaspoon vanilla extract

Procedures

1. Preheat your oven to 350°F (175°C). Lightly grease two ramekins or small baking dishes with coconut oil.
2. In a mixing bowl, combine the mixed berries, 2 tablespoons of maple syrup, lemon juice, ground cinnamon, and ground nutmeg. Toss gently to coat the berries evenly.
3. Divide the berry mixture evenly between the prepared ramekins.
4. In another mixing bowl, combine the old-fashioned oats, almond flour, chopped nuts, melted coconut oil, 1 tablespoon of maple syrup, and vanilla extract. Mix until well combined and crumbly.
5. Sprinkle the oat topping evenly over the berries in the ramekins.
6. Place the ramekins on a baking sheet and transfer them to the preheated oven.
7. Bake for 20-25 minutes, or until the berry mixture is bubbling and the topping is golden brown and crispy.
8. Remove from the oven and allow to cool slightly before serving.

Nutritional Value (per serving): Calories: 250 Kcal, Carbohydrates: 35 g, Proteins: 4 g, Fats: 11 g, Sodium: 2

Peanut Butter Banana Ice Cream

Servings: 2 Prep Time: 10 mins Cook Time: 15 mins Total Time: 25 mins

Ingredients

1 ripe banana, mashed
1/2 cup rolled oats
1 tablespoon almond butter
1 tablespoon maple syrup
1/2 teaspoon cinnamon
1/4 teaspoon nutmeg
1/4 teaspoon vanilla extract

Procedures

1. Preheat your oven to 350°F (175°C) and line a baking sheet with parchment paper.
2. In a mixing bowl, combine the mashed banana, rolled oats, almond butter, maple syrup, cinnamon, nutmeg, and vanilla extract. Mix well until all ingredients are evenly combined.
3. Using a spoon, scoop the cookie dough onto the prepared baking sheet, shaping them into cookie shapes.
4. Bake in the preheated oven for 12-15 minutes, or until the cookies are golden brown and set.
5. Once baked, remove the cookies from the oven and let them cool on the baking sheet for a few minutes before transferring them to a wire rack to cool completely.

Nutritional Value (per serving): Calories: 160 Kcal, Carbohydrates: 30 g, Proteins: 3 g, Fats: 4 g, Sodium: 2 mg, Potassium: 316 mg, Fiber: 4 g, Sugar: 12 g

Servings: 2 Prep Time: 10 mins Cook Time: 25 mins   Total Time: 35 mins

Ingredients

2 ripe bananas, peeled, sliced, and frozen

2 tablespoons natural peanut butter (unsalted)

1 tablespoon unsweetened almond milk (or any plant-based milk)

1 teaspoon vanilla extract

1/2 teaspoon ground cinnamon

Optional Toppings:

Crushed nuts (such as almonds or walnuts)

Fresh berries (such as strawberries or blueberries)

Unsweetened shredded coconut

Procedures

1. In a food processor or high-speed blender, add the frozen banana slices, peanut butter, almond milk, vanilla extract, and ground cinnamon.
2. Blend the ingredients until smooth and creamy, scraping down the sides of the blender or food processor as needed. You may need to pause and stir the mixture a few times to ensure even blending.
3. Once the mixture reaches a smooth consistency, transfer it to a freezer-safe container and freeze for 1-2 hours to firm up slightly, if desired.
4. Serve the peanut butter banana ice cream in bowls or cones, and top with your favorite optional toppings, such as crushed nuts, fresh berries, or shredded coconut.
5. Enjoy immediately!

Nutritional Value (per serving): Calories: 210 Kcal, Carbohydrates: 27 g, Proteins: 5 g, Fats: 10 g, Sodium: 35 mg, Potassium: 470 mg, Fiber: 4 g, Sugar: 12 g

Pistachio and Cranberry Bark

Servings: 2 Prep Time: 10 mins Cook Time: 5 mins   Total Time: 15 mins

Ingredients

1/4 cup shelled pistachios, chopped

2 tablespoons dried cranberries

1 tablespoon unsweetened coconut flakes

1/4 teaspoon ground cinnamon

1/4 teaspoon ground ginger

1/4 teaspoon ground nutmeg

1 tablespoon honey

1 teaspoon coconut oil

Procedures

1. Line a small baking sheet or plate with parchment paper and set aside.
2. In a small bowl, combine the chopped pistachios, dried cranberries, coconut flakes, ground cinnamon, ground ginger, and ground nutmeg. Mix well to evenly distribute the ingredients.
3. In a separate microwave-safe bowl, combine the honey and coconut oil. Microwave on high for 30 seconds or until the mixture is melted and smooth.
4. Pour the melted honey and coconut oil mixture over the dry ingredients in the bowl. Stir until all the ingredients are well coated.
5. Transfer the mixture onto the prepared baking sheet or plate. Use a spatula to spread it out evenly into a thin layer.
6. Place the baking sheet or plate in the refrigerator and chill for at least 30 minutes, or until the bark is firm and set.
7. Once firm, remove the bark from the refrigerator and break it into pieces.
8. Serve and enjoy.

Nutritional Value (per serving): Calories: 160 Kcal, Carbohydrates: 18 g, Proteins: 3 g, Fats: 9 g, Sodium: 2 mg, Potassium: 180 mg, Fiber: 3 g, Sugar: 12 g

Carrot Cake Energy Bites

Servings: 2 Prep Time: 10 mins Cook Time: 5 mins   Total Time: 15 mins

Ingredients

1/2 cup rolled oats

1/4 cup shredded carrots

2 tablespoons chopped walnuts

2 tablespoons raisins

1 tablespoon almond butter

1 tablespoon maple syrup

1/2 teaspoon cinnamon

1/4 teaspoon nutmeg

1/4 teaspoon ginger

1/4 teaspoon vanilla extract

Procedures

1. In a food processor, combine rolled oats, shredded carrots, chopped walnuts, and raisins. Pulse until the mixture is finely chopped and well combined.
2. Add almond butter, maple syrup, cinnamon, nutmeg, ginger, and vanilla extract to the food processor. Pulse again until the mixture starts to come together and forms a dough-like consistency.
3. Roll the mixture into small bite-sized balls using your hands.
4. Place the energy bites on a plate or baking sheet and refrigerate for at least 30 minutes to firm up.
5. Once chilled, the carrot cake energy bites are ready to enjoy!

Nutritional Value (per serving): Calories: 180 Kcal, Carbohydrates: 25 g, Proteins: 4 g, Fats: 8 g, Sodium: 10 mg, Potassium: 250 mg, Fiber: 4 g, Sugar: 9 g

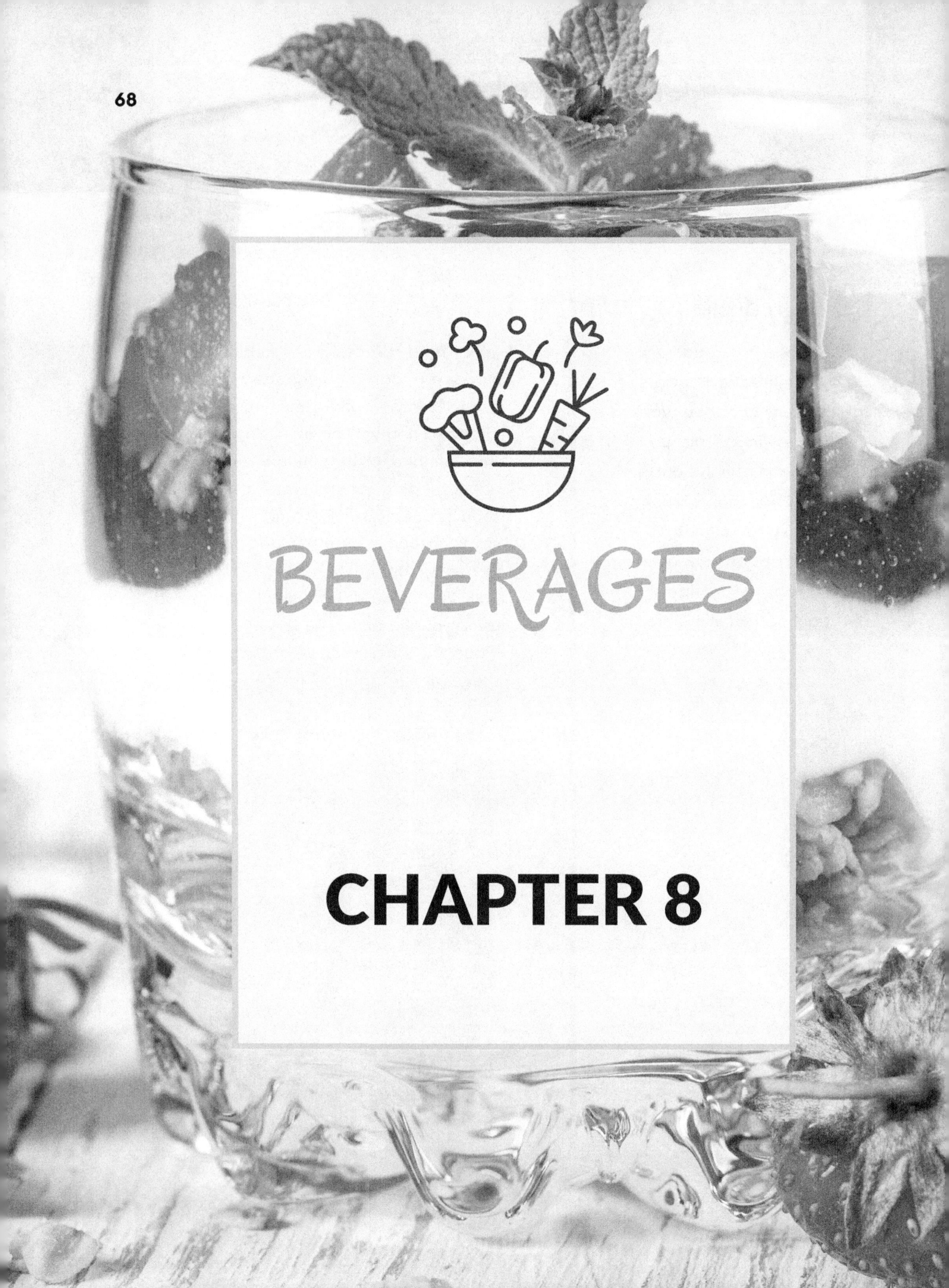

BEVERAGES

CHAPTER 8

Cucumber Mint Cooler

Servings: 2 Prep Time: 10 mins Cook Time: 0 min   Total Time: 10 mins

Ingredients

1 large cucumber, peeled and diced

1/4 cup fresh mint leaves

1 tablespoon freshly squeezed lemon juice

2 cups cold water

Ice cubes, for serving

Fresh mint sprigs, for garnish

Slices of lemon or cucumber, for garnish

Procedures

1. In a blender, combine the diced cucumber, fresh mint leaves, and freshly squeezed lemon juice.
2. Add cold water to the blender.
3. Blend the mixture until smooth and well combined.
4. Strain the mixture through a fine mesh sieve to remove any pulp, if desired.
5. Transfer the cucumber-mint mixture to a pitcher or serving glasses filled with ice cubes.
6. Garnish with fresh mint sprigs and slices of lemon or cucumber.
7. Serve immediately and enjoy.

Nutritional Value (per serving): Calories: 20 kcal, Carbohydrates: 5 g, Proteins: 1 g, Fats: 0 g, Sodium: 3 mg, Potassium: 200 mg, Fiber: 1 g, Sugar: 2 g

Watermelon Basil Cooler

Servings: 2 Prep Time: 10 mins Cook Time: 0 min   Total Time: 10 mins

Ingredients

2 cups diced seedless watermelon

1/4 cup fresh basil leaves

1 tablespoon freshly squeezed lime juice

1/2 teaspoon grated ginger

1 cup cold water

Ice cubes, for serving

Fresh basil leaves, for garnish

Lime slices, for garnish

Procedures

1. In a blender, combine the diced watermelon, fresh basil leaves, lime juice, and grated ginger.
2. Blend until smooth and well combined.
3. Strain the mixture through a fine-mesh sieve into a pitcher to remove any pulp.
4. Add the cold water to the pitcher and stir to combine.
5. Fill two glasses with ice cubes.
6. Pour the watermelon basil mixture over the ice cubes.
7. Garnish each glass with a fresh basil leaf and a slice of lime.
8. Serve immediately and enjoy.

Nutritional Value (per serving): Calories: 60 Kcal, Carbohydrates: 15 g, Proteins: 1 g, Fats: 0 g, Sodium: 2 mg, Potassium: 230 mg, Fiber: 1 g, Sugar: 12 g

Kale Pineapple Smoothie

Servings: 2   Prep Time: 5 mins   Cook Time: 0 min   Total Time: 5 mins

Ingredients

2 cups chopped kale leaves

1 cup frozen pineapple chunks

1 ripe banana

1 cup unsweetened almond milk

1 tablespoon chia seeds

1 tablespoon fresh lemon juice

1/2 teaspoon ground ginger

1/2 teaspoon ground cinnamon

1/4 teaspoon ground turmeric

Ice cubes (optional)

Procedures

1. In a blender, combine the chopped kale leaves, frozen pineapple chunks, ripe banana, unsweetened almond milk, chia seeds, fresh lemon juice, ground ginger, ground cinnamon, and ground turmeric.
2. Blend on high speed until smooth and creamy. If desired, add ice cubes for a colder consistency and blend again.
3. Pour the smoothie into glasses and serve immediately.

Nutritional Value (per serving): Calories: 130 Kcal, Carbohydrates: 28 g, Proteins: 3 g, Fats: 3 g, Sodium: 75 mg, Potassium: 430 mg, Fiber: 7 g, Sugar: 14 g

Mango Lassi

Servings: 2 Prep Time: 5 mins   Cook Time: 0 min   Total Time: 5 mins

Ingredients

1 ripe mango, peeled and diced
1 cup low-fat yogurt
1/2 cup cold water
1 tablespoon honey or maple syrup
(optional, adjust to taste)
1/2 teaspoon ground cardamom
1/4 teaspoon ground turmeric
1/4 teaspoon ground cinnamon
1/4 teaspoon ground ginger
Ice cubes (optional)

Procedures

1. In a blender, combine the diced mango, low-fat yogurt, cold water, honey or maple syrup (if using), and spices (cardamom, turmeric, cinnamon, ginger).
2. Blend on high speed until smooth and creamy.
3. Taste and adjust sweetness if necessary by adding more honey or maple syrup.
4. If desired, add ice cubes to the blender and blend until smooth.
5. Pour the Mango Lassi into glasses and serve immediately.

Cherry Almond Smoothie

Servings: 2 Prep Time: 5 mins   Cook Time: 0 min   Total Time: 5 mins

Ingredients

1 cup frozen cherries

1 ripe banana

1/4 cup unsweetened almond milk

1/4 cup plain Greek yogurt

1 tablespoon almond butter

1 teaspoon honey (optional, adjust to taste)

1/2 teaspoon vanilla extract

A pinch of ground cinnamon

A pinch of ground nutmeg

Procedures

1. Place the frozen cherries, banana, almond milk, Greek yogurt, almond butter, honey (if using), vanilla extract, ground cinnamon, and ground nutmeg in a blender.
2. Blend until smooth and creamy, adding more almond milk if needed to reach your desired consistency.
3. Pour the smoothie into glasses and garnish with fresh cherries or a sprinkle of ground cinnamon if desired.
4. Serve immediately and enjoy.

Cranberry Ginger Sparkler

Servings: 2   Prep Time: 5 mins   Cook Time: 10 mins   Total Time: 15 mins

Ingredients

1 cup unsweetened cranberry juice

1 cup sparkling water

2 tablespoons freshly squeezed lime juice

1 tablespoon fresh ginger, grated

1 tablespoon fresh mint leaves, chopped

Ice cubes

Lime slices and mint sprigs for garnish

Procedures

1. In a small saucepan, combine the cranberry juice, grated ginger, and chopped mint leaves. Bring the mixture to a gentle simmer over medium heat.
2. Allow the mixture to simmer for about 5-7 minutes, stirring occasionally, to infuse the flavors of ginger and mint into the cranberry juice. Remove from heat and let it cool to room temperature.
3. Once the cranberry mixture has cooled, strain it through a fine mesh sieve into a bowl to remove the ginger and mint leaves. Discard the solids.
4. In a pitcher or large bowl, combine the strained cranberry mixture with sparkling water and freshly squeezed lime juice. Stir well to mix.
5. Fill two glasses with ice cubes and pour the cranberry ginger mixture over the ice.
6. Garnish each glass with a slice of lime and a sprig of mint for an extra burst of freshness.
7. Serve immediately and enjoy!

Nutritional Value (per serving): Calories: 50 Kcal, Carbohydrates: 13 g, Proteins: 0 g, Fats: 0 g, Sodium: 5 mg, Potassium: 50 mg, Fiber: 0.5 g, Sugar: 9 g

Blueberry Lavender Lemonade

Servings: 2 Prep Time: 10 mins Cook Time: 0 min   Total Time: 10 mins

Ingredients

1 cup fresh blueberries

1 tablespoon dried lavender flowers

2 cups water

2 tablespoons fresh lemon juice

1-2 tablespoons honey or maple
syrup (optional, adjust to taste)

Ice cubes, for serving

Fresh lavender sprigs, for garnish
(optional)

Procedures

1. In a small saucepan, combine the blueberries, dried lavender flowers, and water. Bring to a boil over medium heat.
2. Once boiling, reduce the heat to low and let the mixture simmer for about 5 minutes, until the blueberries have softened and released their juices.
3. Remove the saucepan from heat and allow the mixture to cool slightly.
4. Strain the blueberry-lavender mixture through a fine-mesh sieve into a pitcher, pressing down on the solids to extract as much liquid as possible.
5. Discard the solids and stir in the fresh lemon juice. If desired, sweeten with honey or maple syrup to taste.
6. Refrigerate the lemonade until chilled, or serve immediately over ice cubes.
7. Garnish with fresh lavender sprigs, if using, and enjoy!

Nutritional Value (per serving): Calories: 65 Kcal, Carbohydrates: 17 g, Proteins: 1 g, Fats: 0 g, Sodium: 2

DASH Diet Grocery List

GRAINS & LEGUMES:
- _____
- _____
- _____
- _____
- _____
- _____
- _____
- _____
- _____
- _____
- _____
- _____

FRUITS & VEGGIES:
- _____
- _____
- _____
- _____
- _____
- _____
- _____
- _____

FROZEN FOODS:
- _____
- _____
- _____
- _____
- _____

CANNED GOODS:
- _____
- _____
- _____
- _____
- _____

DIPS & CONDIMENTS
- _____
- _____
- _____
- _____
- _____

HERBS & SPICES:
- _____
- _____
- _____
- _____
- _____
- _____
- _____
- _____
- _____
- _____

PROTEINS:
- _____
- _____
- _____
- _____
- _____
- _____
- _____
- _____

WHAT'S COOKING:
- **S** _____
- **M** _____
- **T** _____
- **W** _____
- **T** _____
- **F** _____
- **S** _____

DASH Diet Grocery List

WEEK TWO

GRAINS & LEGUMES:
- ○ _____
- ○ _____
- ○ _____
- ○ _____
- ○ _____
- ○ _____
- ○ _____
- ○ _____
- ○ _____
- ○ _____
- ○ _____
- ○ _____

FRUITS & VEGGIES:
- ○ _____
- ○ _____
- ○ _____
- ○ _____
- ○ _____
- ○ _____
- ○ _____
- ○ _____

FROZEN FOODS:
- ○ _____
- ○ _____
- ○ _____
- ○ _____
- ○ _____

CANNED GOODS:
- ○ _____
- ○ _____
- ○ _____
- ○ _____
- ○ _____

DIPS & CONDIMENTS:
- ○ _____
- ○ _____
- ○ _____
- ○ _____
- ○ _____

HERBS & SPICES:
- ○ _____
- ○ _____
- ○ _____
- ○ _____
- ○ _____
- ○ _____
- ○ _____
- ○ _____
- ○ _____
- ○ _____
- ○ _____

PROTEINS:
- ○ _____
- ○ _____
- ○ _____
- ○ _____
- ○ _____
- ○ _____
- ○ _____
- ○ _____

WHAT'S COOKING:
- S _____
- M _____
- T _____
- W _____
- T _____
- F _____
- S _____

DASH Diet Grocery List

GRAINS & LEGUMES:
- ○ _____
- ○ _____
- ○ _____
- ○ _____
- ○ _____
- ○ _____
- ○ _____
- ○ _____
- ○ _____
- ○ _____
- ○ _____
- ○ _____

FRUITS & VEGGIES:
- ○ _____
- ○ _____
- ○ _____
- ○ _____
- ○ _____
- ○ _____
- ○ _____
- ○ _____

FROZEN FOODS:
- ○ _____
- ○ _____
- ○ _____
- ○ _____
- ○ _____

CANNED GOODS:
- ○ _____
- ○ _____
- ○ _____
- ○ _____
- ○ _____

DIPS & CONDIMENTS:
- ○ _____
- ○ _____
- ○ _____
- ○ _____
- ○ _____

HERBS & SPICES:
- ○ _____
- ○ _____
- ○ _____
- ○ _____
- ○ _____
- ○ _____
- ○ _____
- ○ _____
- ○ _____
- ○ _____
- ○ _____

PROTEINS:
- ○ _____
- ○ _____
- ○ _____
- ○ _____
- ○ _____
- ○ _____
- ○ _____

WHAT'S COOKING:
- S _____
- M _____
- T _____
- W _____
- T _____
- F _____
- S _____

Measurement Conversion Charts

If you want to modify recipes from the "Vegetarian DASH Diet Cookbook" to fit your chosen measuring system, you may use this measuring Chart Conversion.

Volume:
1 teaspoon (tsp) = 5 milliliters (ml)
1 tablespoon (tbsp) = 15 milliliters (ml)
1 fluid ounce (fl oz) = 30 milliliters (ml)
1 cup = 240 milliliters (ml)
1 pint (pt) = 480 milliliters (ml)
1 quart (qt) = 960 milliliters (ml)
1 gallon (gal) = 3.8 liters (L)

Weight:
1 ounce (oz) = 28 grams (g)
1 pound (lb) = 454 grams (g)
1 kilogram (kg) = 2.2 pounds (lbs)

Length:
1 inch (in) = 2.54 centimeters (cm)
1 foot (ft) = 30.48 centimeters (cm)
1 yard (yd) = 91.44 centimeters (cm)
1 mile = 1.6 kilometers (km)

Temperature:
Fahrenheit (°F) to Celsius (°C): (°F - 32) x 5/9
Celsius (°C) to Fahrenheit (°F): (°C x 9/5) + 32

Oven Temperature:
275°F = 140°C
300°F = 150°C
325°F = 160°C
350°F = 180°C
375°F = 190°C
400°F = 200°C
425°F = 220°C
450°F = 230°C

Liquid Conversions:
1 teaspoon (tsp) = 1/6 fluid ounce (fl oz)
1 tablespoon (tbsp) = 1/2 fluid ounce (fl oz)
1 cup = 8 fluid ounces (fl oz)
1 pint (pt) = 16 fluid ounces (fl oz)
1 quart (qt) = 32 fluid ounces (fl oz)
1 gallon (gal) = 128 fluid ounces (fl oz)

Dry Conversions:
1 teaspoon (tsp) = 1/3 tablespoon (tbsp)
1 tablespoon (tbsp) = 3 teaspoons (tsp)
1 cup = 16 tablespoons (tbsp)
1 pint (pt) = 2 cups
1 quart (qt) = 2 pints (pt)
1 gallon (gal) = 4 quarts (qt)

Understanding these different measurements and conversions will help you navigate recipes with ease, no matter where you are in the world.

CONCLUSION

Congratulations, my readers, on wrapping up navigating through the pages of the Vegetarian DASH Diet Cookbook! if you're a longtime vegetarian or someone experiencing the world of a plant-based diet for the first time, your devotion to sustaining your body with clean, heart-healthy meals is incredibly remarkable.

As you've learned within these pages, the Vegetarian DASH Diet provides a tasty and sustainable way to reach maximum health. By accepting the concepts of the DASH Diet while including tasty plant-based products, you've taken a proactive step towards increasing your well-being and energy.

Let's take a minute to recall the highlights of our gastronomic visit together:

- We studied the foundations of the DASH Diet and how it smoothly combines with a vegetarian lifestyle.
- We dived into important ingredients and kitchen gadgets to help your culinary ambitions.
- We designed appetizing recipes encompassing morning delights, fulfilling soups and salads, healthful main courses, nourishing side dishes, tasty snacks and appetizers, enticing sweet treats, and refreshing drinks.
- We gave real ideas for success and even supplied an example 3-week diet plan and grocery list to kickstart the preparations.

But our journey doesn't finish here! As you walk into the kitchen to mix up these wonderful delicacies, remember to infuse each recipe with your distinct flare and originality. Experiment with diverse taste combinations, appreciate seasonal vegetables, and most importantly, relish every step of the cooking process.

Did you value your experience with the Vegetarian DASH Diet Cookbook? What dishes did you find most enjoyable? Your input is vital, not just to me but also to other vegetarians seeking inspiration on their own culinary experiences. If you appreciated what you discovered inside these pages, I would be truly grateful if you could write a review and share your opinions. Your feedback will help share the pleasure of plant-based cooking and motivate others to begin on their path towards vibrant health.

Thank you for joining me on this savory and fulfilling trip. May your kitchen always be full of laughter, love, and the aromas of delicious, heart-healthy food.

Here's to your health and happiness, now and always!

Peggy R. Morgan, RDN

Printed in Dunstable, United Kingdom

71845958R00047